SOUL

STEPPING

TEN *Divine* GAMES
TO PLAY WHILE *Walking*

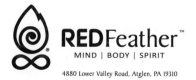

REDFeather™

MIND | BODY | SPIRIT

4880 Lower Valley Road, Atglen, PA 19310

Other Schiffer Books on Related Subjects:

Barefoot Wisdom: Better Health through Grounding
Sharon Whiteley & Ann Marie Chiasson, MD
ISBN: 978-0-7643-5544-8

Designed by Jack Chappell

Type set in Ambient/Merienda/Trajan/Minion

ISBN: 978-0-7643-5719-0
Printed in China

Published by Red Feather Mind, Body, Spirit
An imprint of Schiffer Publishing, Ltd.
4880 Lower Valley Road
Atglen, PA 19310
Phone: (610) 593-1777; Fax: (610) 593-2002
E-mail: Info@schifferbooks.com
Web: www.redfeathermbs.com

For our complete selection of fine books on this and related subjects, please visit
our website at www.schifferbooks.com. You may also write for a free catalog.

Schiffer Publishing's titles are available at special discounts for bulk purchases for
sales promotions or premiums. Special editions, including personalized covers,
corporate imprints, and excerpts, can be created in large quantities for special
needs. For more information, contact the publisher.

We are always looking for people to write books on new and related subjects. If
you have an idea for a book, please contact us at proposals@schifferbooks.com.

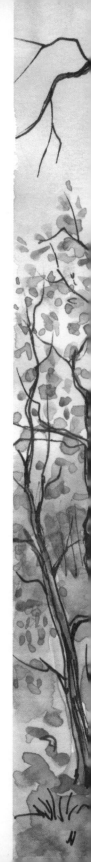

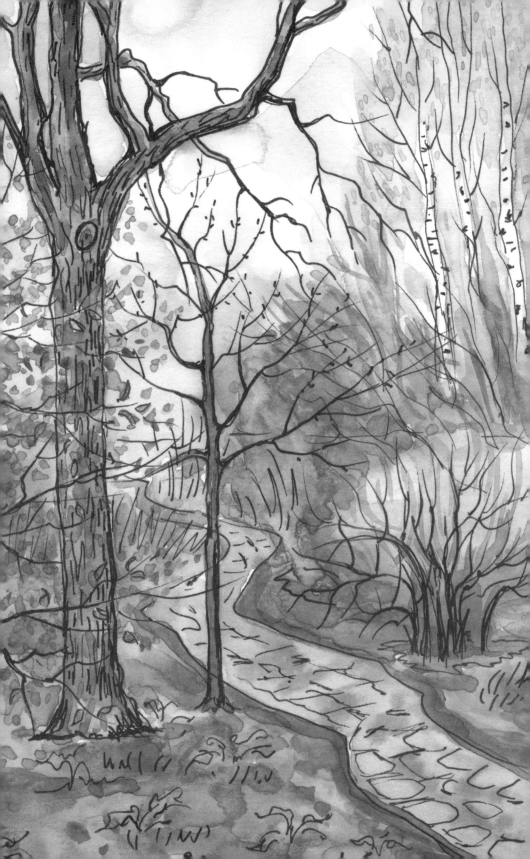

DEDICATION

~ FOR MY FATHER ~

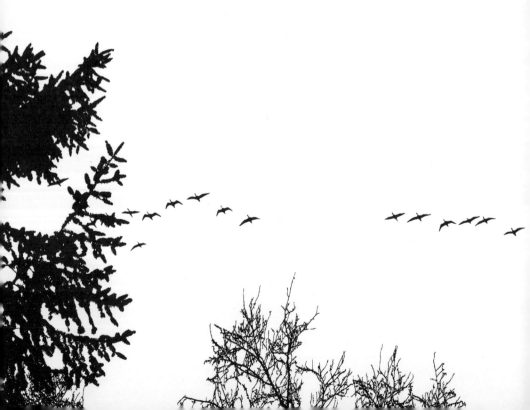

THAT LUMINOUS PART OF YOU THAT EXISTS BEYOND PERSONALITY—YOUR SOUL, IF YOU WILL—IS AS BRIGHT AND SHINING AS ANY THAT HAS EVER BEEN. . . . CLEAR AWAY EVERYTHING THAT KEEPS YOU SEPARATE FROM THIS SECRET LUMINOUS PLACE. BELIEVE IT EXISTS, COME TO KNOW IT BETTER, NURTURE IT, SHARE ITS FRUIT TIRELESSLY.

—GEORGE SAUNDERS

~ CONTENTS ~

～ FOREWORD ～
BY DR. JOE VITALE

I love this book!

What a joyous reminder that the simple act of walking not only is good exercise, as well as a good meditation, but also is a great way to step into the rhythm of your soul and of the Divine.

I love the way the stepping-stone process is taught in this book because it makes it a no-brainer to want to get up and move, as well as a simple way to help manifest more of what you want, or let go of the baggage you no longer want.

I love that the process is a spiritual walking method turned into a game. How cool is that? Now walking has multiple benefits and is fun multiplied.

And I love that there are rhymes that you can sing as you move. It's so much more enjoyable and entertaining to walk and say lines such as these:

> I see. Abundance is a part of me.
> All good comes to me, Easily and continuously.
> All good things come my way. All good things are here to stay.

I also love that this wonderful book includes ways to forgive, as well as ways to create, change your past, attract abundance, get answers, and more. The chapters are easy to follow and well written, and they actually motivate you to get up and out.

Thoreau, Muir, Rumi, and other great "soul steppers" would approve of this book and urge you to read it and practice it. As they knew and taught, walking is a path to your spiritual essence, and that path begins as you walk through the open door.

I am grateful to the author for writing this book, and delighted for you as you are about to embark on a "soul stepping" trek into your own deeper connection to All That Is, or what I often call "The Great Something."

Expect Miracles.

—Dr. Joe Vitale
Author of way too many books to list here!
Visit: www.MrFire.com

~ PREFACE ~

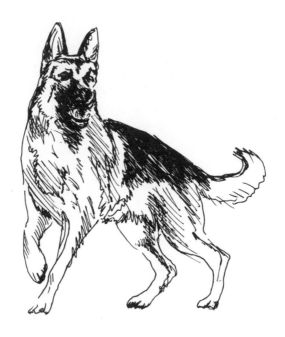

My father considered a walk among the mountains
as the equivalent of churchgoing.
—Aldous Huxley

When I was a very young girl, perhaps ages five, six, and seven, I used to walk with my father. Never the streets, always in the woods. We had miles of forest behind our house. Where the grass ended in the yard, an old, abandoned pipeline began, and from there, the trails into the woods. I never questioned, "Where are we going?" That was never the point. I just walked with my dad. The dogs and I would have followed him to the moon.

Even though I was just a child, I recall being very alert. I listened to the sounds of nature and to my father's voice. We never talked about what was on our minds. We talked about the trees, always checking on their health, looking for rot. And about the birds. He knew the names of them all. We watched for rabbits. I thought I could wish them into being. I can distinctly remember the magic and joy I felt when one jumped out ahead of us. He told me about the history of the land, and once we found an arrowhead. I still have it.

He certainly did not lecture, and yet he gently instilled in me the gift of reverence for nature, animals, and the land.

My father died when I was eight years old. In the first few years that followed, I remember running, grief stricken, my German Shepherd on my heels, up to the paths in the woods. I think now, I must have been looking for him, or traces of him. I wanted to remember. I wanted nature to comfort my broken heart and answer the question "Why?"

I didn't know it then, but what I was doing, while seeking solace among the trees, was inviting a partnership with nature. And she responded. She took me in, wrapped me in her arms, and held me close.

This was a time when it wasn't necessary to keep a constant eye on the children. The forest was safe.

Many years later, when I had children of my own, I reminded my mother of the hours I had spent in the woods, alone. "You had the dog with you," she said.

When I was in my thirties, a time when our early history sometimes resurfaces to be examined, I used to quip that in my childhood I had gone from daddy to dogs. And this was actually true. But also, I realized much later, my father had showed me something else I could go to. When I needed it the most, I returned to walking in the woods.

~INTRODUCTION~

It is not talking but walking that will bring us to heaven.
—Matthew Henry

Imagine you could easily walk away from all of your problems. What if you could put on your shoes, go outside, take a hike around your neighborhood, and come back knowing exactly what to do? How empowering would it be for you to know that you could lift yourself out of depression or anger in the time it takes to walk around the block?

The simple act of walking, literally putting one foot in front of the other, can take you down the road to self-empowerment. You can bring

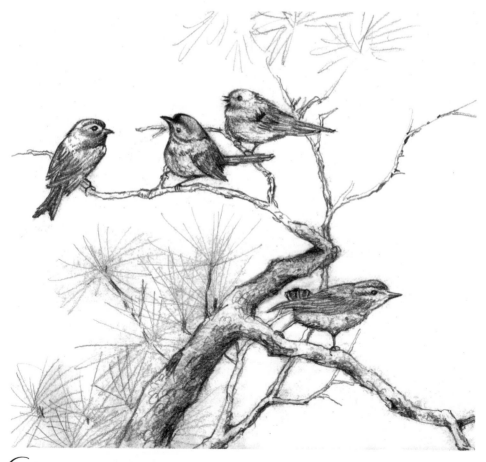

more peace, trust, happiness, and harmony into your life by using walking as your tool. Walking can enable you to answer challenging questions and gain meaningful insights. Walking can transform a lower vibration of depression, grief, or anger into a feeling of calm.

Soul stepping is a spiritual walking method. It is walking with purpose and intention. Soul stepping is a bridge between your physical body, your mind, and your spirit. It can unleash the wisdom and power that is already within you. Soul stepping inspires you to form a partnership with your environment and with nature. It can help you understand the energetic connection your soul has to the natural world. It will deepen your innate intuitive abilities. It can provide all your answers and solutions. Soul stepping is a physical practice that will walk you down a path toward your spiritual and emotional freedom.

The secret is turning the walk into a game.

Tried and tested over the course of three decades, these walking games were derived from my own life experience. What began over thirty years ago as a morning routine to relieve stress soon gave birth to playing what I called "walking games" with myself. I stumbled upon an incredible and reliable resource to obtain answers, or to release myself from the grip of anger or grief. Results were far greater and much more predictable than any other method I had practiced. By using my physical body as a vehicle to let go of my stress, I found I could tap into my spiritual wisdom. I found a way to release all of my struggle and my need to control. And it was easy. And fun.

I offer you ten soul stepping games that you will play with your soul self. By soul self, I am referring to your spirit, to the higher, energetic power in you. Your soul is the vital, divine, intuitive, and sacred self in you that is a part of source energy. It is your connection to nature, to divine guidance, to divinity, to God. It *is* God.

Throughout the book, I may refer to your sacred soul self as God, source energy, or divinity. The terms are interchangeable. I would advise you not to get distracted by specific words or names. Instead, think of your soul as the highest of authorities. Be willing to entertain the idea that there is an all-knowing source energy within you. Whether you acknowledge your soul by a specific name or not, there is an incredible amount of wisdom and power inside of you, ever available, just waiting to be called upon. Soul stepping will help you tap in to your soul and access your all-knowing divinity.

One of the most marvelous aspects of soul stepping is that it is not necessary for you to have a specific faith or a theological background. Anyone can do this. Soul stepping is a spiritual method available to any person, in any walk of life, whether one is a city or cabin dweller. The games can be walked at sunrise on a quiet bike trail or down a crowded sidewalk to the local coffee shop during a lunch break. In most cases, fifteen or twenty minutes is all you need. Unlike an exercise regimen, the games can be played almost anywhere, at almost any time, and will fold nicely into any lifestyle or environment.

Before you begin to actively play the games, you should read through the rules. This section lays the foundation for each and every game. It offers practical tips and gives you the groundwork for successful soul stepping. The importance of breathing deeply and setting your intention before each game is discussed thoroughly.

You can use the games daily or just when you have a specific need. Each game has a theme, so you can pick and choose which game suits you in the moment. At the beginning of each game is a list of life situations, or undesirable emotional conditions, that you might want to change. This section is titled "When to Play." You can read down the lists before you play any game. It should be easy for you to know which game will match up with what you are specifically needing or wanting.

For example, you may need to get an answer to a question, or you might be facing a tough decision. You would play the "Ask a Question" game. If you want to let go of negative thinking or a limiting past belief, you could play the "Walk Away" game. If you are wanting to invite more abundance into your life, you would play the "Game of Plenty." If you are looking to improve your health, you might pick the "What's in It for Me" game. To simply release frustration, you would want to play the "Anger Be Gone" game.

Woven between the games, I offer true stories. I have always loved a good story and perhaps love telling one even more. The true stories that I share here are meant to enrich the games. They are subtle reminders that, very much like a challenging jigsaw puzzle, everything in life really does fit together in some fashion or another.

I also laced the book with information I thought might be helpful and insightful for those on a soul-searching path. These bits and pieces are under the title "The Soul Scoop." They are meant to offer encouragement and to provide you with suggestions to live a more soulful life.

In the back of the book you will find plenty of examples of affirmations and short rhymes. A few of the games require them. They are listed in categories and are included to help get you started in creating your own personal versions.

You will also find an alphabetical listing of signs and omens. This can be an invaluable tool, especially in the beginning, for interpreting what you encounter when you soul step. This list will be particularly helpful when you are playing the "Ask a Question" game. The meanings are brief and should act as a guide for you. The list should help you hone your own intuition and prompt you to communicate more effectively with your own soul and with nature.

The "Animal Totems" chapter will help you discover what animals are your birth totems. Animal birth totems are already in your life guiding and assisting you. This section lays the groundwork so you can begin to work with a wider range of animals in your own life.

The illustrations throughout the book are images of animals that have worked with me during the writing of this book. A few appeared encouraging me to begin the book. Some of the animals arrived during the project and then helped me guide the book to closure. Most were with me from beginning to end. In very defined and personal ways, each one individually assisted me. Including images of them through the use of illustrations is my way to honor them. It is my deepest gratitude expressed.

Finally, it should be noted that one of the magical aspects of practicing soul stepping is that the miracles will continue when the game ends. All the benefits that you gain while playing extend into all other areas of your life. Your relationship with your soul and with nature automatically deepens. Once you recognize the language of your soul, communication will get easier. Your intuition sharpens. Synchronicity will occur regularly. Nature and animals will readily become your allies and willingly assist you at all times. Soul stepping is the invitation to all of that and more.

You are about to embark on a soul journey. Expect the unexpected. Expect miracles.

CHAPTER ONE

THE PATH LESS TAKEN

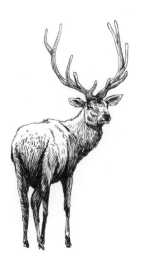

Come, come, whoever you are. Wanderer, worshiper, lover of leaving. It doesn't matter. Ours is not a caravan of despair. Come, even if you have broken your vows a thousand times. Come, yet again, come, come.
—Mevlana Jalal al-Din Rumi

We want to be happy. We look for ways to find relief from our demanding lives. We meet with friends, meditate, and plan vacations. Happiness is the constant search, always the end goal. We think we will be happy when we get the coveted position, or more money, the house addition, or the life partner of our dreams. We hold other people responsible for our own happiness. If only they would change, then we could be happy.

We want more than anything to be free. We strive to maintain stress-free lives. We long for financial freedom. We want a guarantee on good health and long life. We need a little more free time. Often, we feel trapped in circumstances beyond our control. We lash out in unflattering ways or grow despondent like a caged animal, as if we have no other choice.

We react to life as if we are the victims of a cruel plot, as if we do not control our own state of mind.

We have heard the line that "happiness is an inside job," and we may suspect that freedom is too. But often the question remains, "Where inside, exactly?" And once we feel it, how do we keep it?

Soul stepping is a slightly different approach to your happiness and your freedom. You will be walking. You will be using your body to gain access to your soul. Soul stepping offers you a simple way to feel good and also find your answers. It equips you with the empowering ability to tap into your soul wisdom. It shows you the way to help yourself. It can be the journey that leads you to your happiness and freedom.

If you are open and you are even a tiny bit willing, you will discover a wonderful, physical way of working through all of life's challenges. Your soul is waiting for you to call upon it. As you seek your soul, your soul is also seeking you. And it doesn't matter who you are or where you have been, happiness and freedom is just one thought, one emotion, one step away.

When we approach life in a playful, easy way, we can gain understanding and acceptance to our challenges that cannot be accessed through struggle. If we engage the physical body in activity while directing our thoughts specifically, it is possible to unleash the spiritual guidance and the intuition of our souls. To take a walk on purpose, with a clear and specific intention, is to step into a powerful position within your life. Walking in this way strengthens the soul's muscle, taps you into the divine, and will increase the ability to find what you need, when you need it. It's fun, and it's free. You just have to walk out the door.

CHAPTER TWO

ONE STEP FORWARD, TWO STEPS BACK

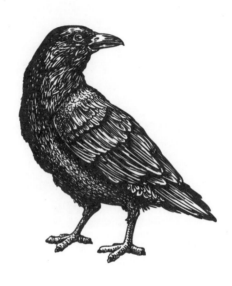

I only went out for a walk and finally concluded to stay out till sundown, for going out, I found, was really going in.
—John Muir

I began a vigorous walking regimen in the late 1980s, when walking was not a celebrated way to exercise. In fact, it was apparently so rare to see someone walking around that people often stopped their cars and would ask me if I needed a ride. Aerobics and running were the exercise fads at that time. It would only be a few short years, however, until walking came into its own right as a valid and effective form of exercise. In the 1990s, walking was actually considered to be one of the most popular ways to exercise. But I did not start walking to exercise. I started walking to save myself.

I first took up walking as a serious endeavor in my early twenties, as a young and busy mother. I was a full-time stay-at-home mom to two children very close in age, and I worked part-time on the weekends. Managing all aspects of the home and my children was an active undertaking. I was fully and completely responsible for my children's needs and their well-being. I juggled the finances and paid the bills. I cleaned the house, cooked all meals, did all the laundry, ran all the errands, and kept the pets happy. Even as I write this now, decades later, I wonder how I did it all.

Making a home for my family and being with my kids 24/7 made me happy, but truth be told, it was challenging and stressful. I was always very, very busy. It was impossible to slow down because there was always more to do. Every single day was packed to the brim with chores and endless activity. I didn't get a whole lot of sleep. My days were generally satisfying, but I often felt like I was running on empty.

I was no stranger to spirituality, and I had more than a passing interest in the mystical and divine. Raised Roman Catholic, I had attended Catholic school and came from an Italian family steeped in faith and superstition. My mother and my aunts had impressive and varied psychic abilities. They often rotated Friday nights between bingo and fortune telling. I knew how to invoke the Blessed Mother and the saints when I needed help. When I got scared, I got down on my knees and prayed. When I wanted to see a glimpse into a future outcome, I read my Tarot cards. If I needed comfort, I read my Bible. To calm my mind and combat my stress, I did yoga for exercise. But I still collapsed at the end of the day, spent and emotionally drained.

At that time, I was a devoted student of the Edgar Cayce material. Edgar Cayce was called the "Sleeping Prophet" because he would lie down on a couch and fall into a trance. In his trance state, he connected with universal consciousness. He gave readings on everything. He recommended cures for disease of the body. He told people about their past lives. He had knowledge of astrology and could access information on the lost city of Atlantis. And he never took a penny for his services. His readings were transcribed, and eventually a hospital and a library were built in Virginia Beach, Virginia. I had used many of Cayce's remedies on myself and my children with much success. And I still do.

The famous psychic often recommended walking. He claimed that walking was the best exercise, and much easier on the joints than running. He highly recommended walking for general well-being and for balancing one's entire system. Well-being and balance was exactly what I was looking for at that time in my life. Cayce offered a rhyming recipe for living a healthy and happy life that served as my inspiration:

"After breakfast, work awhile.
After lunch, rest awhile.
After dinner, walk a mile."

It would be impossible for me to follow the advice exactly. But just the idea of taking a walk every single day was so appealing to me. Thoughts of walking stirred up childhood memories of hiking in the woods with my father. I was drawn to it emotionally. It seemed like such a simple thing to do.

So when my second child entered kindergarten, I put myself on a walking program. In the early mornings, the three of us would walk to the bus stop. When the bus pulled out, I headed down the road.

This was a new juncture in my life—my youngest starting school. I was proud we had gotten this far, but it was emotional to watch that bus pull out with my children onboard. I felt as if I was releasing them into the hands of the unknown. And yet, I craved some peace of mind, some quiet, and a little time for me. I wanted that well-being and balance that Edgar Cayce promised.

There is an old saying about yoga, that some people stay for a class and some stay for a lifetime. The same is true of walking. It can be very addictive, and I soon got hooked. Walking inspired a sense of freedom that had been eluding me for some time. When I walked, no one could account for me, and strangely, the idea of being unaccountable was intoxicating. I would meander down the road at a strolling pace or power walk if I felt ambitious and time was a factor. But in the beginning, it was that feeling of freedom that truly seduced me.

Not long after I made walking a morning ritual, I started to notice that when I walked, my thoughts slowed down considerably, and I became present to the moment. This phenomenon was a fine little break from worry and my cluttered thoughts. I realized my mental thought patterns were often negative. I seemed to be stuck either projecting into my future moments or repeating scenarios of what had already happened. Walking, quite naturally, brought me into the moment of now.

I would often repeat Cayce's catchy rhyme while I walked. The rhyme was easy to remember and fun to say. Sometimes, I found myself singing it under my breath, like a short tune. The rhyme itself would keep my thoughts so concentrated and focused that I would return refreshed and clear headed.

It was my true first glimpse at the wonders contained in walking.

I walked every day, no matter what. I couldn't stop. On the weekends, I brought the kids out with me. They rode their bicycles, and I adjusted my pace to accommodate them. I discovered that walking did, in fact, increase my well-being.

And so my love affair with walking officially began. I walked in fields with my beloved dogs until they got too old to keep up. I walked in the rain and bitter cold. I became an expert, of sorts, on how to dress in inclement weather and still be comfortable. I took great joy in my assortment of raincoats, hats, scarves, and gloves.

I subscribed to *Walking* magazine. I educated myself about dopamine and endorphins, but it didn't take me years to notice that there was something more than the release of hormones going on within me. I started to really listen to my body. I learned to pay attention to my own inner soul urgings. I began to trust walking. More importantly, I began to trust myself.

A little note of caution: Walking will bring out your best and your worst. Like a type of moving therapy, all the garbage, as well as all the gems, will rise to the surface. As I walked, subtle clues about my personality would shine through like small, precious diamonds. I would examine each one individually, as if I was a scientist. I discovered what motivated me and what held me back. Long-forgotten memories from my childhood, both good and bad, would pop into my consciousness. Walking gave me the opportunity to mull them around uninterrupted. Often, after reviewing some incident from my past with adult eyes, I was able to easily suspend a previous judgment. It became easy to release wounded feelings that I had held on to for years. Many times, I would return from a thirty-minute walk with a completely different attitude about a negative past event. I made friends with forgiveness.

I used my walking time like an excavation dig on myself. A previously bolted inner door flew open. I was able to actually listen to myself talking to myself. Soon, I could spot negative thinking patterns and long-held false beliefs. I could hear all the old stories I told myself that ran like broken records. It became enjoyable for me to listen to them. Challenge them. Try to change them. That was my happy walking story for several years.

Then, in 1998, my mother was diagnosed with breast cancer, and she began the fight of her life. Within days of diagnosis, she was scheduled for surgery. I felt like a time thief, stealing the minutes to walk in the predawn before the sun rose above the horizon. My hours at the hospital, and all that came afterward, threw my life into chaos. My housework was neglected, phone calls couldn't be returned, and drive-through happy meals became dinner more often than I like to admit. Stacks of mail that resembled a volcanic science project piled up on the kitchen table unopened. I was doing a juggling act with my family that felt unsustainable. It left me in a constant state of stress, worry, and exhaustion. During my mother's illness, taking the time to walk in the mornings became a mighty challenge. I would often struggle with guilt as I laced my shoes.

My internal dialogue would go something like this: "Can I spare this time? Am I being selfish? I should be doing this task or doing that chore instead. What if I get to the hospital too late and miss the doctor? What about the dishes, the kids, the house, the groceries, my mother, the time . . . the time . . . the time."

Yet always, my wiser, more connected, inner soul self would win over my feelings of worry and guilt every time. I knew from a deeper place that I handled my life better when I took the time, even a brief twenty minutes, to walk. I knew too that once I arrived at the hospital, I would feel trapped, scared, and helpless. Walking was my life preserver in the current sea of chaos and uncertainty. I was aware that when I walked, my emotion of guilt or fear would morph into a type of calming, moving stillness. All I had to do was take those first steps and walk away.

Ironically, it was during my mother's bout with stage 4 breast cancer that I formally started to play walking games with myself, and then with God. The games began as a way to shush the negative voices of the "selfish me," the "bad daughter," "the stressed-out mom," "the lousy housekeeper." Until that point in time, my walking explorations, which had resulted in my various insights and revelations, were quite random. I would simply start walking, and wherever my mind led, like a puppy, I just followed. It wasn't until my mother's cancer and the very real possibility that I might lose her that I deliberately began walking with intention and clear purpose.

And so the games began. One day, I would use the entire walk to pray for my mother. Another day, I might have a conversation with God and express my fears for her life, as well as for my own.

I found I was not ashamed to make bargains with God. In fact, shame itself became an emotion that I abandoned completely. I worked out old wounds and hurts. I healed buried "mother issues" that shockingly bubbled up from the deep and caught me off guard. On several occasions, I listed all the things I loved and appreciated about my mother. Sometimes, I silently repeated mantras, or positive affirmations, that would induce a walking meditative state. I recited Bible verses and poetry that I had learned as a child. Surprisingly, a forgotten line or verse would be remembered, if I stopped struggling and casually let it go. I learned it was a waste of time to struggle. I would ask for signs from nature and then get them.

I became so intrigued with my little games that I started to experiment in a serious and concentrated way. Over and over, I would get marvelous results, or answers to questions, or eliminate an angry or hopeless mood, or gain insight into a problem. I started to rely on them.

My games continued long after my mother's miraculous recovery from breast cancer. I walked right into the years that brought her other cancers and through the final loss of her. Now, when faced with a challenge, a question, a bad mood, or even an unexpected request for my time, my first inner instinct is to "walk on it."

~ CHAPTER THREE ~
TAKING THE HIGH ROAD

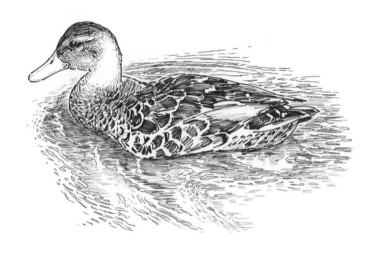

Walk as if you are kissing the Earth with your feet.
—Thich Nhat Hanh

The walking games hold secrets. You can be confident that you will unlock the door to their gifts. Rest assured that your soul has all the information that you will ever need. Your intention is a key.

Dr. Masuro Emoto believed that human thoughts, words, and our intention could alter the molecular structure of water. In the 1990s, Emoto conducted extensive research to prove his theories. Positive, loving thoughts or words directed at a glass of water produced beautiful and dazzling water crystals. Hateful words or thoughts made ugly and deformed crystals. For practical purposes, he believed we could actually change our drinking water with words, thoughts, and intention. We could then benefit when drinking the charged water, and his proof was in the microscopic slides. But can you still benefit by drinking water if you don't direct positive thoughts into your glass? Of course. The benefits of drinking water are inherent in the drinking of it. Many benefits of consuming water, such as hydrating ourselves, for instance, have nothing at all to do with the experiments of Dr. Emoto. Yet, how much more we can profit by the common act of drinking water, if we are aware of the power of our own thoughts and intentions. The power is in directing your intention.

Much like the water experiments of Dr. Emoto, walking can change you, simply with your intention.

You will experience many advantages by walking, because like water, walking has inherent benefits. You will burn calories, reduce stress, and strengthen your body. But by playing the games, much more will be revealed to you. When you soul step, with intention, miracles can unfold.

I have solved pressing problems, answered puzzling questions, calmed the storms of my anger, soothed debilitating grief, received true communication from nature, and been given startling blessings, just from taking a walk. When you intentionally engage the body and consciously and playfully direct your thoughts, you will give birth to amazing results. Walking is a fun, natural, and easy spiritual practice that can offer peace where chaos existed, bring presence to a cluttered mind, and give you the answers that you seek.

Remember, it is not necessary to have a specific religious faith or particular spiritual belief to play these walking games. The games will work for you regardless.

Allow yourself to realize the possibilities. You can drink a glass of water and hydrate yourself. Or you can drink a glass of water, hydrate yourself, and bring more love and happiness into your body and your life. You can take a walk, burn a few calories, and cross exercise off your list. Or you can take a walk, exercise, burn calories, and have real communication from your soul. It's really up to you.

Think about connecting more deeply to your soul as a way of coming home. You have been traveling down this road of life, going down one path or another, maybe making a few detours along the way, certainly hitting a pothole or two. But all along, no matter which twist or turn you have taken, you've really been just trying to get home. Soul stepping is a road map home. Your soul intimately knows you. It has all the answers. More importantly, it is pure divine love and it loves you. It *is* you! The real you. It's home. Walking is one sure way to reach your soul. Soul stepping will bring forth an intimate connection with your soul self and provide a direct line to all the information that it holds.

Soul stepping is a spiritual practice, for sure, but your intention should be to relax and have fun with the games. Answers and insights often arrive more easily when we loosen up and enjoy the ride.

Soul communication is personal. Your soul communication will be unique to you. Most likely, you will not hear a loud voice coming from the sky. The soul is fond of whispering. You may get an intuition, an idea, or a feeling. Often the body will respond to your spirit by giving you goose bumps or chills.

Sometimes just having a bad mood lifted, or a negative belief eliminated, will change your circumstances, and therefore your life, completely. The soul may communicate to you by providing coincidences, a sense of awe, a feeling of relief or deep gratitude, or a true sense of knowing that all is well. Nature is a material manifestation of spirit and will rejoice when you soul step, often providing clear and extraordinary signs and omens. Soul communication always feels good.

When soul stepping, every little thing matters. No thought, idea, feeling, sight, sound, or circumstance will be random. The more you soul step, the deeper the connection becomes and the stronger the trust. Eventually, you will have no doubt that your soul loves you and is eager to assist you in all aspects of your life.

You can read this book cover to cover and then pick a game that applies to a current life situation. Or you can flip through the game titles and choose a game that is just right for a specific mood or crisis in your life.

No one game is better than the other—they all work. You may decide to try all the games in the order that they are listed. Some games will resonate with you immediately, and you will get quick and maybe astonishing results. You may find that two or three games will be favorites and are so effective for you that you use those games over and over again.

Other games might need to be played several times before you feel comfortable with them. I advise you to keep an open mind.

There may be a game or two that you might think you will never play. You'll know them when you see them. When you read the title or the "When to Play," you might physically clench up or feel an inner tug of resistance. I suggest you try them anyway. It is quite likely that the games you find yourself avoiding may be the ones that will benefit you in ways you may not be consciously aware of. These may be the games that will bring about the biggest changes and revelations in your life.

Consider this book as an invitation to play. Allow yourself to let go, to do it for fun, to experiment. Be willing to trust that you already have all that you need. Adopt a light and easy approach and entertain the possibility that everything you need to know will be revealed to you.

A TRUE STORY

When I was nineteen years old, I started doing yoga. As research for a paper I was writing in a Psychology 101 course, I signed up for a six-week class. The class was small, maybe eight people. Everyone there was taking it for a different reason. Of the attendees, I was the youngest in age by at least two decades.

The postures were easy for me. I was, after all, not even twenty. I was healthy, and I had the flexibility of youth on my side. The white-haired instructor was another story. She was well into her late sixties but seemed young and vital. She demonstrated all the poses with ease. She appeared calm and contained. She had been doing yoga since *her* twenties. There was a certain grace and silent happiness about her that I greatly admired. I left class relaxed, yet strangely energized. I wrote my paper, got an A, and signed up for another six weeks.

My yoga interest and practice continued. I read several books on yoga. My favorite, and still a classic, was *Yoga, Youth and Reincarnation* by Jess Stern. I eventually learned enough that I could practice every morning on my own.

When I was in my mid-twenties, I took a random yoga class from a woman named Myra. As it turned out, she would become something of a yoga guru to me over the next three decades. I often joked that Myra ruined you for any other yoga class, because no other class would ever again measure up to hers. Her classes were very different. She stressed the spiritual side of yoga, the "yoking" of the mind and body. We meditated at the beginning and end of each class.

Over the course of the next thirty years, I would fall in and out of attending class with Myra. But every day, I did my yoga. I developed a routine of sorts, doing the same routine almost daily, with the postures that I loved the most. If I felt myself going into what I called "a yoga rut," I would take a class or two with Myra and refresh myself on some of the postures I didn't normally practice or necessarily like.

I once mentioned to Myra my resistance to certain postures and my penchant for getting into a yoga rut at home. Left alone in my practice, I favored some postures and avoided others. She gave a hearty laugh. She said, "Ann, those postures that you are resisting are the ones you need the very most."

Of course, she was right. I felt the truth of her words deep inside myself. From that moment on until this very day, I pay attention to the postures I am resisting. During my practice, if I feel an intuitive nudge to do a posture that I am not wanting to do, I will do it anyway. I have found that it is not so difficult to push a little resistance out of the way. Long ago, I got into the habit of later looking up the benefits of that specific posture. Always, it proves to be just what I need.

CHAPTER FOUR

THE RULES OF THE GAME

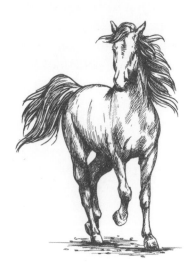

She had headed towards town aimlessly, looking for the kind of escape that could be found only in a solitary walk through a crowd.
—Jade Chang

A true bonus of doing the walking games is that you will get all the surface rewards that a committed walking routine offers. You will burn calories and tone your muscles, and you might shed a few pounds. You will gradually get in touch with what your body says—what your body wants. You will feel better overall and face your days with more balance, well-being, and confidence.

But, the real secret of walking is in *using* the walk to soul step. Adding intention and inviting soul communication while walking is what will bring you the deeper rewards. Your soul will provide answers, help you get to the root of your problems, and give you reliable guidance to move forward in your life.

Start a love affair with your divinity, with your soul. Meet your soul everyday or as often as you can. The more you put your heart into your soul, the more you will direct your energy toward your intentions and the better the results.

Below are a few guidelines and the rules to the games.

SHOES

Always wear athletic shoes. If, for instance, you are playing a game on your lunch break, take a minute to slip into a walking shoe. It is important to be able to walk in comfort and safety.

In addition to being a practical first step, the very act of putting on your walking shoes can trigger the proper mindset for the games. Do it mindfully. Putting on your soul stepping shoes with attention and anticipation sends the brain/body/soul a signal that you are ready to begin. Done often enough, in a ritualistic way, this simple walking preparation will snap you into a present-moment alertness that readies you for soul stepping.

WALK ALONE

The walking games are designed for you alone. Soul stepping is a private and solitary endeavor.

The one exception to this rule is the Gratitude Games. They can be played alone or with friends and family. I have done those games with up to four people. When played with others, the Gratitude Games are hugely beneficial, as well as great fun. When expressing gratitude, the more the merrier.

PICK A PATH

Depending on the game and your state of mind, you may want to give some thought as to where you will be walking—a nature path, a park, a hiking trail, or down the block. Most games you can confidently walk right out your front door. Other games, you may decide to travel to a park or walking trail. This is a personal choice and should not deter your practice of walking. However, if you are always walking down the neighborhood street, you may begin to feel gentle soul tugs to go to a more secluded area where the natural world is more abundant.

In 1995, I read a bestselling book on mindfulness by Jon Kabat-Zinn titled *Wherever You Go, There You Are.* His title has become a catch phrase for me throughout the years and a potent awareness reminder. It aptly applies here and is a truth you cannot escape.

Tape this powerful mantra to your fridge . . . wherever you go, there you are.

BREATHE

Before you actually take those first steps, stand still, get quiet, and take two or three long, deep breaths. Actively engage your senses. Listen to your inhale and exhale. Feel the breath moving through your nose and down into your body. You can do this with your eyes open or closed.

Breathing long, slow, and even will center and ground you. Your breath is a manifestation of your soul. It is truly your life force in motion. By becoming aware of your breath, you acknowledge your soul's very presence. By directing it deeply and slowly, you invite the soul to speak. Listening attentively to the sound of your breathing sharpens your ability to hear the language of your soul. Think of yourself as a conduit for messages. Whisper hello to your soul. Invite its power and guidance into your walking experience.

STATE INTENTION

Finally, state your intention. Speaking your intention out loud, even in a whisper, pulls it out of you. Speaking broadcasts your intention into the universal energetic field.

Your intention is a statement of what you intend to gain during the walk. Be really clear. Make it personal, but frame your intention in a way that empowers you. Words are thought manifestations. The words you speak will set energy into motion. Avoid disempowering phrases such as "I want" or "I need," which tend to keep you stuck in wanting and needing. Instead, use "I intend" or "I choose." When you are asking a question and wanting an answer, begin your intention with words such as "Guide me" or "Show me." State your intention with the expectation that you will get exactly what you need. Believe that help is right around the corner and that your questions will be answered.

There is one of two ways to decide your intention. Let your current life situation determine which game you will play. This will make the intention obvious. Or you can first choose a game that you feel drawn to, and let the game help you mold the intention.

SPECIFIC EXAMPLES:

You've received a new job offer but you are not sure if you should take it. You want to get specific messages that will reflect a yes or no answer. You choose the "Ask a Question and Get an Answer" game, so your intention might be "Is it in my best interest to take this new job?"

Maybe you had an explosive fight with your best friend, so you pick the "Anger Be Gone!" game. The intention could be "I intend to change this foul mood I am currently in and to feel better after this walk." Or simply, "I choose to release these angry feelings."

EXAMPLES OF A STATED INTENTION:

- I intend to connect with my soul.
- I intend to feel healthy and strong.
- I choose to release my worry/fear/anxiety/anger.
- Guide me to the right answer.
- I intend to gain insight on _____.
- I intend to get a "yes" or a "no" to my question _____.
- I intend to appreciate my abundance.
- I choose to let go of this limiting belief.
- Let inspiration guide me.
- Let creativity guide me.
- I will discover what is holding me back.

- I intend to see more clearly concerning _____.
- I choose to heal this current relationship.
- I intend to gain clarity as to why I am experiencing this current physical symptom/illness.
- Show me a sign that my angels are with me.

There may be times when you are in such an emotional state that you don't even know what you want. But the truth is, we always want something. It is there; we just have to put it into words. The very fact that we are experiencing a heightened negative emotional state is the evidence that we are not getting something that we want, even if it is just peace of mind. Feeling emotional turbulence is often the moment when actually speaking your intention will be the most powerful. You first need to ask yourself, "What do I want?" The answer to that question might be "I just want to feel better." So your intention could be "I intend to feel better." Or simply, "Help me."

In her book *Traveling Mercies*, Anne Lamott expressed my own private sentiments by saying her most used prayers are "Help me, help me, help me" and "Thank you, thank you, thank you" (Lamott 1999). In the time of your darkest emotions, often the most basic and sincere words can act as the perfect intention.

Hold your intention and begin walking. Believe and trust that you are walking toward your answers.

BE CONSISTENT

The games are available for you to play when you need them—when you are in a crisis, you need to make a decision, you are depressed and can't shake it. But by playing daily, or at least a few times every week, you will strengthen your connection to your spirit. Soul communication will become more identifiable and prominent in your life. You will learn your soul's language. You will begin to recognize your soul's messages, prompting you with guidance as intuitive hits or nudges. Most definitely, your intuition will sharpen. If soul stepping becomes a habit, the natural world will begin to respond to you in amazing ways. Because you will be deepening your connection to nature, you may notice that animals show up more consistently demanding your attention.

The soul loves to be invoked and appreciated. Your soul will continue communication after the game has ended. The games will act as a catalyst to awaken an awareness in your consciousness, like a domino effect. You will begin to understand that everything is connected. Your outer world is a reflection of your inner world. There are no random events. You will begin to notice coincidences, and divine synchronicity will lovingly unfold as you move into your days. Your dreams may become more vivid or prophetic. You may start to experience more abundance and unexpected financial opportunities, especially when you make the "Gratitude Games" a regular practice. People whom you encounter may begin to say the words that are just what you need to hear. Life can begin to take on a magical quality, as you rely more and more on the guidance you receive and cultivate a trusting relationship with nature and with your soul.

You should keep in mind you will often get immediate and startling results. But not always. Sometimes the results will be subtle, and you will have to dig a little deeper and be consistent. For instance, if you have been stuck in the same old victim story for forty years, you will get very good results with the "Change Your Story" game the very first time you play. But for long-lasting and permanent change, you will need to play it several times.

You may notice that you feel drawn to playing certain games over again. Listen to your intuition. Enjoy the sense of relief at the end of the walk. Notice how the positive emotions you feel during the games extend into the rest of your day. Expect to see satisfying changes in your experience when you play the games consistently.

LET GO

Letting go is a guideline that will ultimately free you. The spiritual practice of letting go of control can be slippery and is often contradictory. We long to surrender, yet we grasp so tightly to our agenda, to our victim story, to our to-do list, to our point of view. In the case of soul stepping, letting go means trusting. Really trusting. It means surrendering to your higher power. Letting go is accepting the guidance and the answers that you receive, even if they are not the answers that you want. Letting go is about suspending judgment. It means not manipulating or predicting the results. It means relax, just let go of the reins, and allow the experience to carry you.

Let go of being attached to the outcome. Being attached to an outcome is wanting to control an outcome. The need to control is rooted in fear. Clinging to a specific result implies that the universe doesn't support you. It blocks other possibilities that may be far greater than you can imagine.

Attachment to outcome is a mental habit that you can change. The trick in changing mental thinking patterns is to first become aware that you are doing it in the first place. Listen to the thoughts you are thinking. Replace fear-based thoughts with new thoughts. If done repeatedly, you can cultivate a new belief that everything will turn out for your highest and greatest good. Be vigilant. When I catch myself clinging to a desired outcome, I use a miracle phrase that will snap me out of it immediately. I tell God, "You take it from here."

Believe that what you need will show up, sometimes in startling and stark ways, sometimes in a subtle whisper, sometimes after the walk is over.

A TRUE STORY

I have loved horses my entire life. There were farmers on my father's side of the family, so I had exposure to them at a young age. Like many little girls, I dreamed of someday having horses of my own.

For various life reasons, my own horses never materialized. And so it was that in my forties, I decided to officially take riding lessons.

During my lessons, I always rode the same horse, Sugar. I was inexperienced, but earnest. She was gentle and forgiving. I fell head over heels in love with her. Over the course of several weeks, as I grew more confident in my skills, we established a mutual trust.

One day we were on a long ride through the forest. Sugar was sure-footed, the autumn weather was perfect, and I was happy. My instructor was riding in front. About midway through the ride, she told me that a little farther up the trail, we would be crossing a creek. She said Sugar wasn't fond of water and might get a little nervous. But the creek was very shallow . . . a trickle. Nothing to be concerned about. Sugar has crossed it before, she said—just move her through and she would be fine. My thoughts raced. What? Sugar doesn't like water? Move her through?

Sugar heard the water before I did. Her ears went forward, her muscles tensed a bit, and her pace slowed. I knew I was in charge. That she would take her cues from me. But I couldn't help it; I was getting nervous too. We got to the creek and Sugar stopped. She took a few steps back. I told her we could do this, although now, I didn't really believe that we could. I did my best to move her through. She wouldn't budge. She would back up, I'd get her going forward again, and then she'd freeze. We carried on this way for several minutes. My instructor was up ahead, stopped, and was watching all of this.

I was embarrassed. It was pretty obvious who was leading whom. I had all these lessons under my belt and had felt fairly confident, until I was up against a true test. I told myself that I should be able to get this beloved creature through a trickle of water. It was *my* lack of trust in my own ability, *my* nervous energy perpetuating this situation, and I knew it. I tried to relax and muster control, but you can't lie to a horse.

Finally, my instructor said stay put, and she would dismount and walk us across. "No. No. I got this," I said, but I saw her getting off her horse. Okay then, I thought, if that's what it takes. It is what it is. I want to cross the creek. It doesn't matter how we do it. I took a mindful deep breath and just let go of all resistance. I suddenly felt a shift of energy. Before I could even settle into the feeling of my surrender, Sugar jumped across the narrow creek! To my own astonishment, I stayed on her. And there we were, not through, but over.

In that moment, this white horse became one of my greatest teachers.

That exhilarating experience was a potent reminder for me to trust and to let go of preconceived notions of how situations *should* be. Again and again, like a patient instructor, life will reinforce that all really is well.

~ CHAPTER FIVE ~
THE GAME LIST

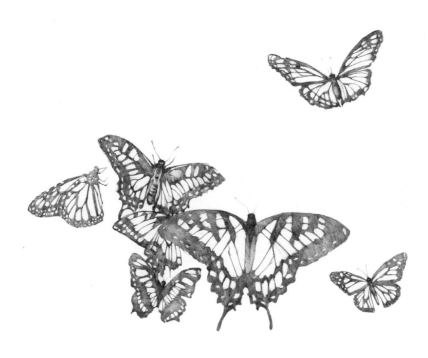

Pursue some path, however narrow and crooked, in which you can walk with love and reverence.
—Henry David Thoreau

Here are ten of my best walking games. I regularly use the following games with unfailing results. You will get results too. For each and every game, remember to first take a few deep breaths and set your intention.

Each game has a different theme and is targeted for a different kind of result. Some games are geared toward bringing you specific answers. Other games will aid you in shifting your vibration, help you release resistance, and put you in a better-feeling soul space. The advantages of feeling better should not be underestimated. Often, reducing the intensity of a bad mood might be exactly what is needed to bring a change to your situation. Soul stepping helps you quickly process and naturally shift your thoughts and feelings in a healthy and timely way.

To assist you in choosing the right game for the right time, there is an array of life situations and emotional reactions listed under "When to play." Read through the lists and play the games that fit your particular circumstance.

The minimum suggested time for most games is twenty minutes. Twenty minutes is recommended for you to fully realize the benefits for each game; however, the time can be adapted to your specific need. You may see marvelous results in just ten minutes. Depending on the game, and your specific circumstance, you may choose to walk for forty minutes or more. Make it work for you and have fun doing it.

I want you to think of soul stepping as first establishing, then deepening, a connection to your soul. It might help to imagine your soul as a new friend or lover. Put your best foot forward. Get to know each other. Have a few experiences. Enjoy each other. As your relationship deepens, so will your trust, and eventually you will come to rely on the insights, information, and blessings that you will receive.

~ GAME ONE ~
THE BIG EMPTY

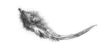

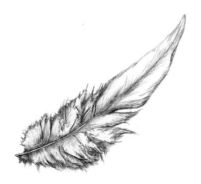

RELEASE MENTAL CHATTER AND BECOME PRESENT.

I walk regularly for my soul, and my body tags along.
—Sarah Ban Breathnach

TIME: 20 MINUTES OR MORE

WHEN TO PLAY:

- You feel as if your life is out of control.
- You feel overwhelmed.
- Your mind is cluttered.
- Your environment is cluttered.
- You want to inspire new ideas.
- You feel depressed.

- You are bored or in a rut.
- You experience worry, fear, or anxiety.
- You feel you never have enough time.
- You are experiencing dissatisfaction with life.
- Life is too busy and going too fast.
- You are mourning the loss of a loved one.
- You feel lonely.

HOW TO PLAY:

Take a few long, deep breaths and state your intention. Start out walking at a comfortable pace, and after approximately one or two minutes, just stop. No need to time this with a stop watch. You can judge the time internally. It is not so much about precision timing as it is about calling up your intuition and listening to your soul voice.

While you are standing still, look around. What do you see? What can you hear? What does your body feel like? What thoughts arise?

At the beginning, your mind will actually answer these questions. You will tell yourself, "I see the trees, I am hearing nearby traffic, my hands are tingling, or these shoes are pinching." That's okay. Smile (for real) and listen without judgment to yourself. Attune yourself to what your body is saying. Take note of what your mental responses are when you stop. Are you appreciating, complaining, or just noticing without judgment? How does your body feel? Are you more aware of your body or the thoughts you are thinking? Be present and pay attention. All of your reactions are clues.

From here, you will now walk at your normal pace about 40–50 steps, silently counting your steps as you go, and then stop again. Counting the steps forces your mind to stay focused and present. When you stop, you are letting go of the mind's voice that is counting. You are breaking a pattern. Each time you stop, be present. Look around. Engage the senses. Feel your way to the moment. Watch how your thoughts move in and out again. Be alert and aware.

The pause should be at least thirty seconds to a minute, but take as long as you need. Then start moving again. Another 40–50 steps, counting as you go, and again, stop. It is fun to mix up the number of steps, taking 40 at one interval and then 50 or 60 in the next. It will also benefit you if you change the pace of your walk between stops. Walk fast, then stop. Walk slowly, then stop. Let your intuition guide you. It is less important how many steps you choose to take than it is to stay really focused on the counting when you are moving. When you stop, relax, pay attention, and let your mind empty out.

Be very alert to what feelings, thoughts, and emotions surface when you stop. Recall your intention. Your soul may offer a sudden insight. A solution to a problem might occur to you. A long-forgotten memory, good or bad, might surface. Tears may spring forth for no apparent reason. A question may occur to you that you never thought to ask yourself. Whatever happens, happens. Or maybe . . . nothing happens! Just blessed presence. It is all good. Just stay with it, watch it, and then start moving again and count the steps. Pay attention; suspend all judgments. Don't concern yourself with getting it right. You cannot have a "wrong" experience. The emphasis is on *paying attention*.

In short, it looks like this:

Intention . . . walk . . . stop . . . walk and count steps . . . stop . . . walk and count steps . . . stop . . . walk and count steps . . . stop . . . continue.

This walk is about emptying and letting go of the clutter inside. By emptying out, you make space for presence. Emptying will bring you into the present moment and can help you invite a sense of joyful vitality into your experience.

There is a fair amount of yin and yang going on in this game. Fast and slow, start and stop. The true desired condition sought is *balance*. Walking in this way gently nudges your consciousness out of routine and pulls you into the present moment. This game is a good introduction into soul language. It will help you listen more attentively and feel your emotions more deeply. It exercises true listening, so you can better tune into the messages of the soul.

A TRUE STORY

The November morning was unseasonably warm, but breezy. It was the day before Thanksgiving, and tomorrow I would be hosting and cooking dinner for thirteen people. I felt overwhelmed, and I didn't have a whole lot of time to spend on a morning walk.

We had always gone to my mother's house for Thanksgiving. My mother loved to cook, and she enjoyed the large family dinners. But we had lost her two years before. I was experiencing feelings of grief and mourning holidays past. I knew that tomorrow I would have a house full of guests, mostly family, but she would not be there.

I still had a lot to do. There was last-minute cleaning, bringing in extra chairs, and all the meal preparation that could be done the day before. I was capable of accomplishing all of this, of course, but I had a cloud of grief hanging over me that seemed to cover and darken any joy I could experience. Instead, I felt stressed out, and I missed my mom. I needed to empty out emotionally.

My intention for my walk that morning was to release my feelings of stress and grief. I walked, I stopped, I counted steps. It didn't take long before I started to feel attentive and present to my immediate surroundings. I was able to let go of the long to-do list that had been circling and repeating itself in my thoughts. I began to appreciate the autumn colors, the burgundy- and rust-colored leaves. A subtle shift of light seemed to produce a glow on everything around me, and the sheer beauty of the landscape held my attention.

During a stop and pause, I heard a small plane flying above me, and instinctively I looked up and watched it. The sky was filled with cotton candy–type clouds. Everything had a supernatural, reverent radiance, and even the clouds looked angelic to me. As I watched them, the clouds changed their shapes. I could clearly see angelic bodies with heads and wings. In my awe, I remembered a story my mother had told me.

She was riding home after a chemo therapy treatment. She knew within hours she would be very sick. This was a scary time. Still one more treatment and another month before we would know if they were working.

On this day, looking out of the car window into the sky, she saw a single cloud formation. Surrounded by a brilliant blue, the clouds moved into the perfect form of a solitary angel. She saw every detail of the angel clearly and sat frozen in her seat as she watched it smile down at her. Immediately filled with a strong, loving kindness, she had the absolute, knowing awareness, without a single doubt, that she would be all right. She knew that she would get through these awful treatments, that she would live.

And she did live. She was cured of the cancer and lived another twenty years.

She had told no one, but me, this story.

So on that November morning, when I saw the clouds that looked like angels, I remembered my mother's story. My grief melted like snow. I knew she was sending me this sign. She was telling me that she was with me still, and joy filled my heart. By emptying out, I had opened up the space for a message of love.

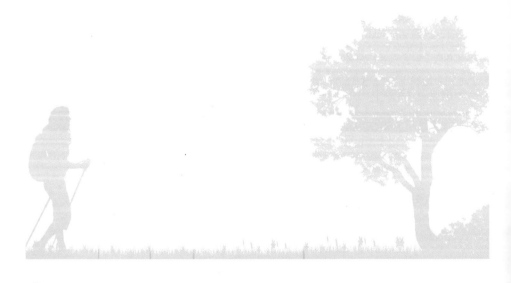

~ GAME TWO ~
GRATITUDE GAMES

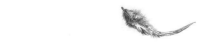

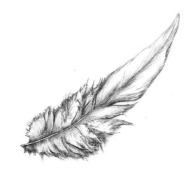

A THANKING FRENZY

THE ABCs OF GRATITUDE

Perhaps the truth depends on a walk around the lake.
—Wallace Stevens

TIME: AT LEAST 15 MINUTES OR MORE

WHEN TO PLAY:

- You are feeling sorry for yourself.
- You feel like a victim.
- You are having frequent arguments with friends or family.
- You want to manifest a desired outcome.
- You feel like something is missing in your life.
- You are having financial fears or worries.

- You are bored or in a rut.
- You feel as if there is lack in your life.
- You are depressed.
- You feel hopeless or powerless.
- You feel like nothing is right in your life.
- You have a creative block or need new ideas.
- You are experiencing chaos in your life.

A THANKING FRENZY

HOW TO PLAY:

Take a few long, deep breaths and state your intention. Begin walking at a comfortable pace and start "thanking." You can thank silently or out loud. Thank everything you see, everything you feel, everything you hear. Thank your surroundings. Thank your body, your mind, your soul. Thank your friends and your enemies. Thank your blessings and your curses. No breaks in your thanking thoughts are allowed. Thank throughout the entire walk in a nonstop, continuous manner.

At first, it will go something like this: "Thank you, trees. Thank you, sky. Thank you, birds. Thank you, arms. Thank you, legs." But as you keep moving along, because the game requires you to keep thanking without breaks, you will notice your gratitude expanding. What started out as you saying words to simply say something will deepen into true, vibration-shifting gratitude. Your "thank you, legs" will soften and expand into "thank you, legs, for carrying me through my life. Thank you for making this walk even possible."

Think of gratitude as a soothing and magical elixir that has the power to heal everything it touches. Allow the vibration of gratitude to grow and grow, until it permeates your entire being.

THE ABCs OF GRATITUDE

Take a few long, deep breaths, and state your intention. Begin walking at a comfortable pace, and use the alphabet, starting with A and ending with Z, to name things you are grateful for. Truly grateful for. State the letter and then a grateful match to the letter. Much different than "A Thanking Frenzy," you may need to think for a minute before you say something. For example, you may say, "A. I am grateful for ants." But are you? What about those carpenter ants in your kitchen this spring? Are you grateful for them? I would hope so, but if not, you can't use it. Maybe instead, you could say, "A. I am grateful for apples!" You have to mean it. The game is not about matching words to the letters of the alphabet and intending to make your gratitude fit those words. It is about making the letters and words fit your gratitude.

Continue through the entire alphabet.

The ABCs game is an adaptation of an Abraham-Hicks process that I heard Ester Hicks recommend. When I first heard the process and tried it out, I loved it. Playfully practicing gratitude produces such profound shifts in vibrations that I wanted to include my own soul stepping version here. When I added soul stepping and the "gotta mean it" rule and reached for real gratitude with every single letter, the results were enormously satisfying. When we move the body while expressing gratitude, it opens blocked energy channels and we can release resistance. As you continue walking and moving, you will find joy and gratitude naturally bubbling up to the surface.

Either gratitude game is a good choice when you are short on time and only have a few minutes. They will also work like soul medicine when you are feeling out of sorts, a little blue, or just need a quick pick-me-up. Expressing gratitude is a fast and effective way to shift your energy.

Both games can be played alone or with other people. Group gratitude is not only fun, but you receive the added energy lift that is the result of combining forces. If you play the ABCs game with one or more other players, you will take turns with the alphabet. Someone starts with the letter "A," the next person gets the letter "B," and so on back to you, through the entire alphabet.

My daughter and I have played gratitude games in order to curb an argument or when we've felt our conversation getting tense. It has never failed to return us into a balanced and loving state of mind.

Several years ago, all of my female cousins met at Virginia Beach for a getaway vacation that we coined the "Cousins Reunion." We all got along just fine and were having a great time, and there was a marvelous, easy flow to our days. But one morning, having stayed up late drinking wine on the beach the night before, we couldn't seem to come to agreement about the plan for the day. One of us wanted no plan, another wanted to go eat breakfast, and another wanted to get to the beach before the midday sun became unbearable. Up until this particular morning, no one seemed to mind which way any day went. Any suggestion was a good suggestion, and we had managed to effortlessly please everyone. So on this morning, I suggested we do a little gratitude soul stepping and bring back that easy flow. Only the smallest amount of encouragement was needed. Soon we were walking the sandy shore and thanking our lucky stars. In a few short minutes, we were laughing, our energy lifted, and we were having so much fun that everyone forgot their own agenda. Afterward, we felt restored, took a swim, had breakfast, and then lounged around for an hour and told family stories.

When we are in a place of appreciating, of relishing what we already have, of exaggerating our existing bounty and blessings, we attract more to appreciate and relish. The universe always says yes. Gratitude elevates our vibrational frequencies because it is an expression of love. When we send out signals of love and gratitude, the universe responds by sending us more to love. Practicing gratitude lifts us out of resistance and struggling mode and puts us into receiving mode.

Do not underestimate the raw power of gratitude. It can be life changing.

CLEARING CLUTTER

My dated, and well-thumbed, *Webster's Dictionary* defines clutter as "a number of things scattered in disorder." In the ancient Chinese practice of Feng Shui, the definition broadens to anything that is not used, wanted, or loved. It also includes spaces that are overcrowded, even if the area appears to have order. All physical things are made of energy. Too many things in a room or house can block the flow of energy.

We are affected by our surrounding spaces physically, mentally, and spiritually. An overcrowded room equals energy that can't move. Cluttered spaces will make us feel stuck, cranky, and fatigued. It can stop the flow of abundance, financial or otherwise. Stuffed spaces will contribute to stuffed-up noses or clogged sinuses. If neglected long enough, cramped and crowded areas can start to slow down circulation and will eventually break down the bodies vitality. In a nutshell, physical clutter will wreck havoc in your life and on your body.

Mental clutter is just as dangerous. Frenzied mental activity, a tendency to worry, negative thinking, feeling overwhelmed, and not being able to prioritize tasks are signs that we may need some mental and physical housecleaning. Mental chaos will eventually manifest as physical clutter in our environment. The outer is always a reflection of the inner.

Spiritual pursuits will often take a back seat when our space and our mind are cluttered. Stagnant energy in a space makes it difficult to experience a sense of awe, peace, or calm. It is hard to practice mindfulness, meditation, or any spiritual practice in an overcrowded room.

In a sly way, clutter also robs us of time. We waste time looking for things. When we have so much stuff, our things get buried and forgotten. Often, we go out and purchase items we already have.

Physical chaos also has symbolic connotations that cannot be ignored. Messy desks can be a reflection of dissatisfaction with work. An overstuffed purse, or a wallet in disarray, can indicate financial strain. A front doorway that is a disorganized drop for mail, coats, shoes, and bags can not only block new opportunity from entering but shows an unwillingness to fully engage in life.

Purging clutter is good for the body and for the soul. It creates space and movement and frees up energy levels and blocks. Clearing clutter benefits our overall health and state of mind.

To begin clearing clutter, it is a good idea to start out small. Tackle your purse, a single drawer, one cabinet, a pileup of paperwork, or your desk. Even small clutter-clearing efforts will open energy flow and can create movement in specific areas of your life. As a Feng Shui practitioner, I recommend starting in an area or direction that represents what is currently blocked in your life. Having money or debt issues? Start with your wallet and look at clutter in the southeastern part of the home. Work problems? Clean up the desk. Check in the northern part of the home or anywhere paper and mail accumulate. Experiencing poor health? Look at the center of the home and the bathroom. Make sure hallways are open and not blocked. Is your romantic relationship suffering? Begin in the bedroom or southwestern part of the home. If you are not sure where to begin, the front-door area, where opportunity enters, is always a good choice.

When you are clutter clearing and feeling attached to certain items, there is a simple rule of thumb to follow. Ask yourself: Do you use it, do you need it, or do you love it? If not needed or being used, then you should love the item. If it's not loved, get rid of it.

Duplicate items, or things not currently used or needed, might fall into the "I might need it someday" category. This attitude reflects the fear of lack. It sends out the vibrational assumption that you will not be abundant in the future. In this case, ask yourself: "If I was moving, would I take this?"

When you are letting go of your items, a good mindset to adopt is an attitude of gratitude. This practice is often forgotten in the clutter-clearing process. Feeling grateful can help you let go of things that have outworn their usefulness. When you appreciate how your items have served a purpose in your life, it becomes easier to release them. Gratitude will actually create space for you mentally and physically. When we are grateful, we feel full and abundant. Gratitude generates feelings of generosity and makes it easier to give. It helps you realize when you have more than enough.

Thank the items that you are releasing. They have served you in some way. Offer gratitude to your things, bless them, and then donate, sell, or give them away. Donating an unwanted item allows another person to use it and love it.

A CLUTTER-CLEARING TIP

When my mother passed away, I faced the overwhelming, emotional, and daunting job of cleaning out her house. Although my mother kept a tidy home, she had lived there for over fifty years. She was also very sentimental, and she had saved a lot of things.

Six months went by, and I was not even half the way through. During a phone conversation, I told a girlfriend how those months had gone by so quickly. For all the time I had put in, I didn't feel like I was making much progress. She listened, and then she gave me an invaluable tip. She said to set a timer for one hour and work for only one hour. If you go over the hour, consider it a bonus.

I really liked this idea, although I didn't think it was very practical. There was still so much of the house to go through. I feared that this task may take me years if I worked there only for such a short time. But putting in only an hour at the house felt like a relief. I wanted to give it a try.

So, every evening, I went to my mother's house and set her stove timer for one hour. Immediately, I saw results. Because I wanted to make the most of the one hour, I got started right away. No more dillydallying around. If I found something that stopped my progress, such as love letters my father had written during the war, I'd sit on the floor and read the hour away. But when the timer went off, I got up, and I went home. Many more times, I charged through one hour and then two, and then maybe three.

Since then, I have used this one-hour tip for jobs both big and small. Sometimes, I use it when there is a lot to be done in a single day. I break the different tasks into one-hour segments.

This tip is an amazing and unsurpassed clutter-clearing tool. Clutter bust in one-hour sessions. It is a doable time frame with a clear-cut beginning and end time. You will be astonished at how much can be done in one hour.

~GAME THREE~
ANGER BE GONE!

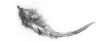

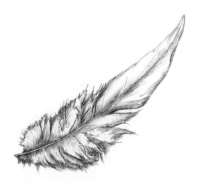

TRANSFORM ANGER TO CALM.

It is impossible to walk rapidly and be unhappy.
—Mother Theresa

TIME: 20 MINUTES OR MORE

WHEN TO PLAY:

- You are angry or enraged.
- You have been betrayed.
- You feel frustrated.
- You are overwhelmed.
- You are in a bad mood.
- You want to experience more joy in your life.
- You had an argument with someone.
- You feel resentment.

- You feel envy.
- You are experiencing dissatisfaction with life.
- You find it difficult to forgive.
- Something has upset you.
- You are mentally replaying an upsetting situation that occurred.

HOW TO PLAY:

Take a few long, deep breaths and state your intention. Begin walking at a fast pace. Walk in a marching fashion, as fast as you can. You are not lifting the knees, but simply stepping in a normal way and swinging your arms as you walk. Exaggerate the swinging and stepping motion. Right arm should come up with the left step. Left arm up with the right step. Someone watching would think you were power walking, but the swinging of your arms is not a pumping action. Do not bend your elbows. Instead, keep your arms straight, but not stiff. Your hands should be open and relaxed, not in a fist. You will continue marching rapidly throughout the entire game.

In the first few minutes of the game, focus on your physical body and the marching movement. Keep moving as fast as possible. Notice how your body feels tense with emotion. Use your attention to scan your entire body to see if there is an area that feels especially blocked with emotional energy. Common areas to hold emotions are the chest, stomach, and lower abdomen, but emotion can be held anywhere. If you find a spot that feels tight or denser in the body, mentally pull the energy to your heart center.

After approximately three to five minutes, move your awareness from your physical body to your feelings. Now is the time to allow your emotion to emerge. Identify the emotion that is driving you. For instance, you may say, "I am feeling so angry." Allow yourself to fully feel the emotion.

While still marching, imagine that the area of your heart is the center that contains the emotion that you want to release. Scan your body, and if there is any emotional residue, pull it all into your heart center. Try to feel the emotion as swirling or vibrating energy in that area of your chest.

Next, in your mind's eye, see yourself holding onto a stone. Feel the weight of it in your hand. Now, visualize the negative emotion leaving your heart center as an energy stream and pouring into the stone that you are holding. Name the emotion and declare it gone. "Anger be gone! Jealousy be gone! Betrayal be gone!" Then, mentally drop the stone, still chanting, and leave the emotion behind you. You transferred the energy of your emotion into another form, you dropped it, and now you are walking away from it.

Thoughts may surface that are attached to the emotion. You may find yourself justifying your own position in the form of a story you want to tell yourself. Put the thoughts or stories into stones and drop them. Continue to chant your emotion, thoughts, or stories to be gone. You are walking away from a trail of stones. You are freeing yourself to move forward.

This game is a walking visualization that uses the power of your spoken word.

It is an incredibly effective way to diffuse and release any negative emotion, not just anger. Taking your negative emotion from inside your body and putting it into a stone helps rid you of its impact. When we visualize, the brain does not know the difference between what is real and what is imagined. Using this moving visualization allows you to mentally zero in, break up the energy of the emotion, rid yourself of it, and leave it behind you.

Using a marching step while walking, which is swinging your opposite arm to your opposite leg, will correct energetic imbalances. Walking this way can be used any time you feel out of sorts.

In the world of energy medicine, the marching motion is an effective tool to balance the body's right and left hemispheres. According to author Donna Eden, considered the mother of the energy medicine movement, each energetic hemisphere of our body needs to cross over to the opposite side. Stress, negative thinking, and high-impact emotional scenes can scramble the natural direction of our energetic hemispheres. When our body's energy is moving in the correct way, our brains can operate at peak level, we can process life more efficiently, and our physical body will also heal more rapidly.

A TRUE STORY

Several years ago, there was a woman who walked the streets in my hometown.

The first time I saw her, I was sitting in my car at an intersection, waiting to pull out and eager to get home. It had been snowing for hours and the roads were icy, but I was less than a mile from my house. Crossing directly in front of my car, this woman was walking very determinedly. Her age was hard to guess. She had thinning, white hair that was blowing mercilessly in the bitterly cold January wind. She was wearing an unbuttoned, knee-length winter coat, which was flapping wildly. Absurdly, she was holding an open umbrella out in front of her. Apparently, this was meant to break the wind, although it wasn't doing a very good job. It all appeared so contrary.

I had several fast, first thoughts. I thought it was odd she was using an umbrella to break the strong winds but hadn't bothered to button her coat. She was walking so fast and with such determination that her whole body was leaning forward. She looked as if she was marching to battle. I wondered where on Earth she was going in such a hurry. Did her car break down? I looked up and down the road. I didn't see a stranded vehicle. Should I offer her a ride? But just as I had this last thought, as if she could read my mind, she turned and looked, quite pointedly, directly at me. Her expression was hostile—hateful. It so startled me, it even invoked a bit of fear. No, I did not want to offer the ride. Now, I hoped she kept on going and didn't come up to my car. She did pass and I pulled out. I remained unsettled and puzzled by her. Mental illness, or possibly Alzheimer's, never entered my mind. I was more rattled by the force of the energy she threw at me with her aggressive look.

I started to see her walking all around town that winter. She always walked very fast. She gave the impression that she was in a hurry, determined to arrive. I avoided eye contact.

One day as I was entering the parking lot of a local shop, I saw her walking from the back of the building and turning into the street. When I went inside, I asked about her.

The store clerks had several tales about her. She warns the girls about waiting on the other customers. She claims that they are criminals, sell drugs, or plan to rob them. One clerk claimed that several times the woman had been on foot, standing behind a line of cars in the drive-through lane at the bank.

Now, it became apparent to me that the woman suffered from dementia or mental illness. This brief conversation moved me from initial curiosity to real concern. Does she live alone? Is family taking care of her? No one knew.

About a month later, my son had an encounter with her. He was walking his dog behind his house and saw her walking on his property. Immediately upon seeing him, she began shouting at him that he had stolen this land from her. She was loud and confrontational. He didn't want to engage her in conversation, so he turned and went back down the hill to his house. She didn't follow, but she turned around as well and went back the way she had come. He continued to watch her as she walked back to the road. She opened all the mailboxes and even removed a newspaper from one of them. She opened it, briefly read it, and then folded the paper neatly and politely put it back.

Sightings went on all that winter and into spring. The neighbors talked; a few had called the police out of concern. By midsummer, it became common knowledge that she wasn't homeless, that she lived on the east side of town, and that her son was looking after her.

I sent her silent prayers and quietly wished her well when I saw her walking on the streets. She had proven herself to be harmless, after all, and actually appeared to be rather robust. If she has nothing better to do, I thought, why not walk?

I also repeatedly made an interesting observation. If I saw her close to her home on the east side of town, her face would be tense and contorted with an angry, hateful expression. But if I spotted her far on the west end of town, miles from her home, her face and posture appeared neutral. Her facial features would be significantly more relaxed. I was well aware of the power that walking had to ease troubled emotions. It wasn't a large leap to conclude that after she had walked a mile or two, her anger subsided. The transformation was profoundly reflected in her body language and her face. Walking helped her ease whatever demons she was battling. I hoped that she would be able to continue.

I do not know the ending to this walking woman's story. Deep into the following winter, it occurred to me that I hadn't seen her for weeks. I asked around. Again, no one knew. Because she had family, I let myself assume that she was being cared for. I rested with the knowledge that she had been able to walk regularly and that walking surely had made her life experience a little easier.

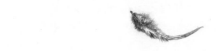

～ GAME FOUR ～
THE AFFIRMATION WALK

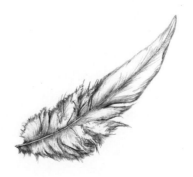

USE AFFIRMATIONS AND MANTRAS TO CHANGE YOUR LIFE.

I wish to walk and keep the ways of God.
—Lailah Gifty Akita

TIME: 20 MINUTES OR MORE

WHEN TO PLAY:

- You are depressed, sad, or unhappy.
- Your mind is cluttered.
- You are overwhelmed.
- You are ill.
- You want to lose weight.
- You are worried, fearful, or anxious.

- You feel as if nothing is going right in your life.
- You want to change your life and yourself.
- You want to break an old habit.
- You want to change negative thinking.
- You want to manifest a desired outcome.
- You are looking for a romantic partner.
- You want to heal a current relationship.

HOW TO PLAY:

Before you begin, choose one affirmation or mantra that applies to your situation. An affirmation is a statement that is used to create a positive change in your life. We use affirmations to change negative thinking and destructive self-talk. Affirmations should invoke feelings of joy and happiness. They are expressions of what you want, but are stated in a way as if it already exists.

Use upbeat and positive words that redirect a negative thought or situation that you are experiencing. Phrase your affirmation in the present tense. Keep the focus of the words on what you wish to create for yourself.

To begin, take a few long, deep breaths and state your intention. Start out walking at your normal pace while repeating the affirmation. Say the phrase over and over—nonstop. Do not break the rhythm of the phrase. You can speak silently or aloud, or both.

The idea is to crowd out all other thoughts for at least twenty minutes. When any other thought enters your mind, gently let it go. Return to repeating your affirmation or mantra and focus on the words you are saying. You may be inclined to go off on a thinking tangent because the affirmation may invoke mental arguments or resistance. Release those thoughts and keep pulling yourself back to the affirmation. Say the words with emphasis and meaning.

The affirmation or mantra will begin to take on a kind of rhythm. You can step in time to the rhythm of your words. In this way you are using your body to put emphasis on the words.

Your soul will bring forth clues about what you are trying to change in the form of emotion. Notice the feelings that your words invoke. Are you feeling more happiness, more joy? Are you feeling resistance, not truly believing the words you are saying? Notice everything that comes up for you, but don't stop saying the affirmation. Do not allow your thinking to catch and keep you. Just notice your thoughts and feelings and gently go back to saying the affirmation.

Often, after five or ten minutes, you will feel as if your affirmations or mantras are just sounds that you are making. They may create a hum within your body. This can be extremely helpful in dislodging old, negative emotions. Sound is healing to the body. Allow your voice to resonate through your entire being. This can induce a feeling of moving meditation. You can play with the tone, beat, and volume of your words. Walking in this way provides a rest for the busy mind and healing for the body. The soul gently guides you into an alert, present state. You will be rewarded with a refreshed attitude and a changed mind.

Speaking positive affirmations over and over helps reprogram conditioned beliefs that may not be serving you. By repeating the words, your subconscious mind begins to accept the new statements as true. If you play this game often, you will notice yourself saying the affirmation throughout the day. Like magic words, they will surface when you need them. Most importantly, you will begin to believe them.

You will find examples of affirmations in chapter 6.

~ THE SOUL SCOOP ~

A STORY

Long ago, in ancient times, there was an unholy man, desperate for repentance.

He called out the name of God repeatedly.

Day in and day out, night after night, he uttered the word.

His tongue swelled. His lips bled.

The Devil heard this plea, and one night he appeared to the man.

"Hey, you stupid man," the Devil said. "Not once has God come to you. You call and call and does He appear? No, there is nothing!"

And the Devil smiled.

The man fell to the ground, more desperate than before.

Exhausted, he went into a deep sleep.

The prophet Abraham appeared to him in a dream.

He asked the man, "Why do you regret calling out to God?"

The man said, "I called day and night. God never came. He did not reply and tell me 'Here I am.'"

Abraham smiled and said, "God has told me to tell you this. 'It is in the calling of my name that is my reply. Your very longing for me is my message to you. Your attempts to reach me are my attempts to reach you! It is in the silence surrounding your every call of my name that I answer, 'Here I am.'"

—Adaptation of a story written by
Mevlana Jalal al-Din Rumi

~ GAME FIVE ~
ASK A QUESTION AND
GET AN ANSWER

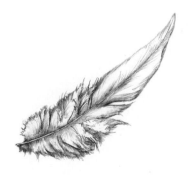

GET ANSWERS TO QUESTIONS.
UNDERSTAND SIGNS AND OMENS.

Look deep into nature, and then you will understand everything better.
—Albert Einstein

TIME: 30 MINUTES OR MORE

WHEN TO PLAY:

- You need an answer to a question.
- You are confused about a situation.
- You are unclear as to what to do next.
- You want to connect to nature.

- You are seeking guidance from nature.
- You need creative inspiration.
- You want to manifest a desired outcome.
- You are experiencing grief.
- You need to make a decision.
- You want a sign or omen about a recent decision.
- You need a yes or a no answer.
- You are looking for better direction in life.
- You are overwhelmed.

HOW TO PLAY:

Take a few long, deep breaths and state your intention. After you have clearly stated your intention, ask nature to work with you. Begin walking at your normal pace.

At the very start of the game, you will want to keep your question in the forefront of your mind. After a minute or two, as you continue to walk, you can allow the question to drift away into the background. Begin to pull your attention to the present moment and become alert to your surroundings. It is important to pay attention to everything! What you see, and what you feel when you see it, will be the answer to your question.

This game is best played in a natural setting. It isn't necessary to drive to a remote mountain path, but the idea is to connect and communicate with nature wherever you choose to walk. You can walk on the road in your neighborhood. A walking trail or a bike path in a local park is ideal. Nature is everywhere and will work with you and respond to your desire to connect.

Even in an urban environment, you can communicate with nature. Pigeons, squirrels, insects, flowers, clouds, even sidewalk weeds can offer insight when you ask and are willing to see. Nature's language is one of symbolism. Pay attention to the natural world around you and notice anything that nature shows to you. Keep track of the small signs as they appear. Nothing is accidental.

THE ENVIRONMENT AND WEATHER.

Notice what happens in the environment around you. Pay attention to the light and any shifting weather patterns. Has the sun come out from behind the clouds, or have the clouds now blocked the sun? Did a sudden comforting breeze just sweep over you? Has it started to rain? Was there a light drizzle when you started out walking and now the sun is shining?

THE TRAIL OR STREET.

Is the walking trail or street clear, or have you come upon an obstacle in your path? Do you suddenly trip? Are you continually having to step over something? Has your way been blocked? Do you see any items on the path, perhaps a feather, a pencil, or someone's trash? Do you find anything? Do you keep it or walk right past? Sometimes items that you normally would not notice will catch your eye. Go ahead and pick up that feather, the stick, or stone when playing this game. Nature might be offering you a powerful totem.

FLORA.

Do you see any flowers or trees? What kind are they? Does a specific color attract you? Do you feel drawn to stop and sit under a specific tree or linger near a bunch of flowers? Follow any urges you may get. Are you seeing only weeds or unattended grasses? Are there wildflowers in the weeds? Do any insects capture your attention?

PEOPLE AND ANIMALS.

Are you alone during the entire walk, or do you come across fellow travelers? Does someone speak to you? What do they say? Are they friendly or do they ignore you? Do you notice groups of people laughing and having a good time? Do you witness an argument? Do you see children or adults or both? What are they doing? What animals or birds do you see? What kind of animal is it, and what is it doing? Are the animals wild or domestic? Does someone have a friendly dog that wags its tail? Does a dog see you and aggressively begin to bark? Or do you not see any animals or birds at all?

THOUGHTS AND FEELINGS.

When you are practicing presence, your soul will have a direct line of communication with your consciousness. Are there thoughts nagging at your awareness? What are they? Did an idea or answer pop into your awareness? Are you fretting or complaining to yourself? How are you feeling? Do your feelings change throughout the walk? Do you have a sudden shift in mood? Did you start the walk feeling anxious about a situation and now you find yourself relaxed and calm? Or the other way around?

Everything that you see, hear, and experience in this game is a message. Every single thing is a gift from your soul and nature. As you continue to play this game and exhibit a willingness to work with nature, you will be awed and amazed at the ease in which your answers come to you. In chapter 7, I provide a list for you to help interpret the signs and omens that you receive.

If you are looking for a yes or no answer, it can come in a multitude of ways. Perhaps the sun came out? A yes. Was the sun out and then clouds blocked it the entire walk? Your answer is likely a no. Did that light breeze give you goose bumps? That was spirit giving you the green light. Did you trip and skin your knee? Your answer is probably a no, because you might get hurt otherwise. You will want to interpret everything on your walk to gain a deeper insight into your question. Approach this game with openness and a willingness to trust, and thank nature for any answer that you receive.

EXAMPLE ONE:

You have received a job offer that would be an increase in salary but also requires you to travel farther. Your current employment is close to home and very secure, but you haven't had a raise in two years. You ask, "Should I take this job offer?"

You start out walking and nothing really happens. You feel anxious about getting a clear answer and have been worried about what to do. After about ten minutes, it gets windy. As the breeze continues to pick up, you start to feel chilly and have to zip your jacket. You notice dark clouds on the horizon, and just then you hear a single crow cry out and see it fly across your path. It startled you, and instinctively you stop for a second and watch it.

The answer to the question is no. The chilly breeze would be interpreted that you will be uncomfortable in the new position. The dark clouds on the horizon would mean the job may bring unfortunate circumstances in the future. The single crow calling out warns you to stop and stay where you are.

EXAMPLE TWO:

You have been dating someone and are wondering if there is a future in this relationship. You are compatible in general and feel you might be falling in love, but recently you have had an argument that made you question if this relationship is going to work in the long term. You ask, "Is there a future with _____?"

You begin walking down the local bike trail and immediately have a feeling of relief. It just feels good to be outside and walking. The sun is out and the day is beautiful and warm. Although you started with a serious question, you soon find your thoughts relaxing. Your thoughts drift to a memory of a dinner date you had last week with your partner. You remember something funny that was said, and it makes you chuckle out loud. You see young squirrels playing and chasing each other up and down a large, old oak tree. A little later, you hear someone talking behind you and glance back to see a couple riding bikes. You walk to the side and let them pass. It is an elderly couple, and they both smile and say hello.

Your answer to the question is yes. The beautiful day, the comfortable weather, and the feeling of relief confirms the satisfying nature of the relationship. The happy memory and chuckle puts the current argument into perspective, and now you want to laugh it off. The squirrels playing suggests that even fun-loving relationships have ups and downs. The old oak tree indicates a good, solid foundation for the relationship. The friendly older couple predicts a happy and easy union in the future.

It may take a little practice to understand and interpret the nature messages, but it is well worth the effort. The more that you are willing to receive the guidance from nature, the easier interpreting will become. The guide at the back of the book will be helpful for you. But always trust your own intuition.

Walking in this way will cultivate trust between you, your soul, and nature. Your soul will never lie to you. Nature will never lie to you. You may not always get the answers that you want, but soul stepping will always provide the truth.

A TRUE STORY

My good friend Betsy was living and working in Ojai, California, and was a manager at an upscale hotel. She liked her work and was making a decent living, but she wasn't truly fulfilled. One day, out of the blue, she was offered an opportunity to manage a private resort in the Grenadine Islands.

The position was quite lucrative. The contract was temporary, only six months. Although she had a close and tightly knit family, her children were grown. She didn't have any current romantic ties. It would be a good time in her life to do this. The sheer adventure of living on an island was alluring and thrilling.

But Betsy was settled in and loved living in Ojai. She had wanderlust but wasn't sure if she wanted to completely uproot her life. She knew if she left that for six months, contact with her family would be at a minimum. Here in Ojai, her family was within driving distance. She also knew that after six months, she would not be able to return to her present employment.

It was a big decision to make. I suggested she take a walk and ask nature.

Equipped with her journal, she headed to a favorite trail just outside Ojai in Los Padres National Forest. Halfway along the trail, as she rounded a bend, she was stopped dead in her tracks by a very large rattlesnake sun bathing in the middle of the path. There was no way around him. The left of the trail was the steep wall of the canyon and to the right was the drop-off.

Betsy was a frequent hiker, but she had never seen any snakes in California. She wasn't fearful, but she knew she had to turn around. On her way back, she stopped and sat on a large rock in the mountain stream. She sat for a while and just listened to the sound of the water.

Hiking out, just before the main road, she encountered another rattlesnake. This snake was in the middle of the trail as well, and rattling!

Betsy stood calmly and waited a very long time. It did get quiet but didn't move. She sent peaceful and nonthreatening thoughts and hoped he didn't have family in the thick grasses and undergrowth on both sides of the path. Finally, making a very wide circle, she walked off the trail.

Betsy realized that as long as she was alert and consciously present to the changes in her life that she would be okay.

In the end, she took the offer and went to the island. It was an adventurous, worthwhile experience for sure, but she did not stay on for a second term. Nearing the end of the contract, she was eager to fulfill her obligation. She felt time was standing still. She was grateful for this opportunity but was beginning to feel isolated. She missed her family.

Snakes means change, caution, and transformation.

The first rattlesnake across the path meant that her life as she knew it would stop and that things would change. There would be no fear of the change, but she would go back and not stay permanently.

On her hike, Betsy went to the water. In this case, she literally did travel to an island surrounded by water.

The second rattling snake appeared right before she could return to her car. She waited a long time and had thoughts of his family. No harm came to her, and she got to her car safely. This, too, played out exactly.

The change and relocation proved to be a bit rattling. Yet, she remained calm and cool. Toward the end, she felt as if she was waiting to get home again. She finished her contract with thoughts of family on her mind.

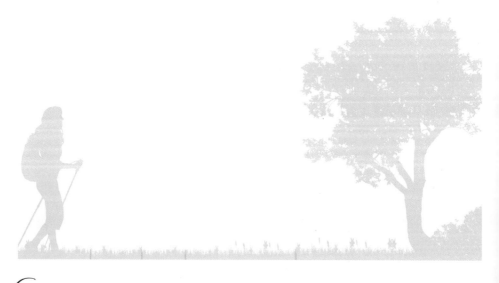

~ GAME SIX ~
THE "I LOVE YOU" GAME

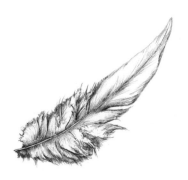

A GAME CHANGER FOR RELATIONSHIPS.

Don't threaten me with love, baby. Let's go walking in the rain.
—Billie Holiday

TIME: 30 MINUTES OR MORE

WHEN TO PLAY:

- You feel disappointed in a relationship.
- Someone has hurt you.
- You are unable to forgive someone.
- You are unable to forget something someone has said or done.
- You had an argument with a loved one.

- An old emotional wound has surfaced.
- You are repeating negative patterns with people in your life.
- You are telling yourself negative stories about someone.
- You are complaining about someone.
- You want to experience more happiness in your relationships.
- You just had a breakup.
- You are getting a divorce.
- You are placing blame on others.

HOW TO PLAY:

Take a few long, deep breaths and state your intention. Begin walking at a comfortable pace and pick up momentum and speed as you go. Toward the end of the game you will be walking briskly.

At the start of the game, bring your attention to the person who has disappointed or hurt you. Think of this person in a general sense. Do not get caught in the trap of repeating a negative incident that happened. Think of this person as someone who is not attached to you. Be generic in your thoughts. In your mind, briefly describe them in a subjective way, as if they were a stranger. For instance, "He is 5'11", has short brown hair, and likes to swim." Keep your emotions out of the description. See them as someone neutral to you. Release any attachments to them. This should not take more than a few minutes.

Then, for the next five to ten minutes, begin to think of them as a child. Recall any details from their childhood that you may know. What did they go through as a child, as a young person growing up? What was their home like? Did they have loving and supporting parents, or not? Did they experience any trauma or loss as a child or young person. Might something in their childhood have changed them or caused them to think and act a certain way? Did they struggle financially? Were they doted upon or barely acknowledged? An only child, or one of many? Did their parents lean toward the negative or the positive?

If you do not know any details about this person's childhood, still think of them as a child. Imagine them as they might have been. This person came into the world as a vulnerable baby. They learned to walk and then to run. They were subjected to parents and an environment they had no control over. Imagine them as the innocent child they once were. If the person is your own offspring, think of them first as your newborn baby. Remember your delight when they took their first steps or said their first word. Call up memories of joy and laughter.

For the next ten minutes or so, begin to tell yourself about the qualities you like about this person. Recall past experiences that were pleasurable. Is there something about this person that makes you smile or laugh? What are the characteristics about this person that you really appreciate? What initially attracted you to this person? What do you love about them? Allow yourself to feel good about this person. Exaggerate the good things. List them one by one. Crowd out any negative thoughts. Keep appreciating. Keep loving.

For the remainder of the walk, hold an image of this person in your mind and begin to say the words "I love you." Say the words nonstop, over and over.

This game is very effective for any relationship issues you have with a specific person. Your thoughts and feelings about this person will shift. You will experience a more balanced and loving emotion within yourself before the game ends.

The game is broken up into four segments: neutral description (five minutes), childhood (five to ten minutes), appreciation (ten minutes), and love (ten minutes.) All parts should blend together seamlessly. I recommend this time frame to use as a guideline, but it is only a guideline. Trust yourself when it comes to how long each section will take. Every situation will be unique.

The soul will naturally and gently lead you to memories and intuitions about an individual that will soften your current feeling toward them. Follow where your heart and soul take you. Any anger, frustration, or resistance that is present is simply an emotion that is produced by your thoughts.

This game is not about giving anyone a pass for bad behavior or abuse of any kind. The game will not change anyone. What this game will produce is a change in you. Bringing love into any situation changes the situation. This game will invite an opening in your heart that will bring enormous clarity. Perhaps the clarity comes in the form of healing discord between two people. Or, when coming from a place of love and understanding, you may choose to end a relationship or peacefully distance yourself from someone.

~ THE SOUL SCOOP ~

HO'OPONOPONO

There is an old Hawaiian healing practice called *Ho'oponopono*. It is pronounced the way it is written, six syllables, all long O's, as in the word "no." At the core of the practice is the basic premise that everything begins with you. You must accept responsibility for everything. If you want anything or anyone in your life to change, you must first change you.

In 2007, author Joe Vitale popularized the ancient practice in his book *Zero Limits*. Prior to writing the book, Vitale searched for, and finally found, Dr. Ihaleakala Hew Len. Dr. Len was known for healing dangerously insane criminals at a Hawaiian hospital where he was employed. Dr. Len helped an entire ward of patients who had been previously all but given up on. The most fascinating thing about the patients' turnaround was that Dr. Len had never interviewed, interacted, or seen any of these people. He used the healing technique of *Ho'oponopono*.

Until *Zero Limits* hit the market, not much was widely known about the practice. However, the basic premise is simple. It involves assuming that anything "wrong" with someone else first starts with you. You simply accept responsibility for it, ask the Divine for forgiveness, inject a dose of love, and top it off with gratitude.

Ho'oponopono offers several methods to accomplish this, but the easiest and most popular one is the repeating of four simple sentences:

"I love you.
I'm sorry.
Please forgive me.
Thank you."

By saying the three magic words "I love you," you are connecting immediately with the Divine within. You say "I am sorry. Please forgive me" as a way to acknowledge that there is a place in you that is responsible.

You accept responsibility. If we are all one, what is in you is also within me. Then the gratitude. "Thank you." It is done, and I am grateful.

Saying these lines in mantra fashion, over and over again, is said to produce healing of all varieties.

It is not a quick fix or magic bullet. It is a practice and requires practice. Wonderful results can be had, however, by saying these lines when you have had a disagreement with someone.

Using these sentences while soul stepping, perhaps after an argument, can change your internal energy and therefore change the entire situation. You can adapt the "I Love You" game to include the other three sentences for the last ten minutes. Walking while declaring love, forgiveness, and gratitude is very effective for shifting, and eliminating, negative emotion. The movement of walking will help break up heavy, condensed emotion and help you shift more easily into feelings of gratitude.

~ GAME SEVEN ~
THE GAME OF PLENTY

SEEK AND FIND ABUNDANCE.

If you are walking to seek, ye shall find.
—Sommeil Liberosensa

TIME: 30 MINUTES OR MORE

WHEN TO PLAY:

- You are experiencing lack.
- You are worried about money.
- You can't get ahead financially.
- You have trouble meeting monthly expenses.
- You are hoarding.
- Your house is cluttered.

- Your mind is cluttered.
- You feel envy.
- You feel jealousy.
- You find it hard to be generous.
- You are allowing bills to stack up.
- You have an unwillingness to deal with your finances.
- You want to live an abundant life.

HOW TO PLAY:

Take a few long, deep breaths and state your intention. Begin walking at a comfortable pace. Look around you. Pay attention to your surroundings. Appreciate everything you see. Notice how abundance is everywhere.

Begin to cultivate a feeling that there is more than enough of everything. Look at the countless leaves on the many trees. Notice the abundance and generosity of nature. Look at the unlimited openness of the sky, the vast expanse of the very land that you are walking on. Think of the ocean and the grains of sand on the shore. See the wonder and immense abundance in all that is nature. Imagine all the countless insects, birds, animals, and people in the world.

Now, make abundance personal. Start to think of the abundance in your life that is already present. Can you count how many pairs of shoes you have? How many rooms are in your apartment or house? How many windows? How much food is in your refrigerator, freezer, or cabinets? Can you name all that is there? Try. How many items of clothing do you have hanging in your closet? How many towels are in the bathroom? How many *things* do you actually own? Start naming them.

Next, move your thoughts of your things to your body and your life. How many hairs are on your head? How many beats does your heart take in a day? How many breaths will you take on this walk? How many steps? How many words do you speak in a single hour? How many emotions pass through you in a day? How many days have you already lived?

Really acknowledge that you are already living with abundance. You already have plenty in your life. You should begin to have a subtle sense of "fullness," as if you just completed a satisfying meal. You should feel relaxed and contented.

As you are finishing up the game, ask your soul for a sign today that more abundance is coming into your life. Offer gratitude and say thank you, as if it has already arrived. Sometimes, immediately, you will find a coin or a natural token from nature, perhaps a feather. Maybe as the day moves forward, someone gives you something. You might see a rainbow while driving. Be watchful and expectant throughout the day and there will be a sign given to you. Know that your source is continuously providing, tirelessly replenishing, and constantly giving.

The idea is to realize, and begin to know, that true abundance is a feeling. When we feel abundance and gratitude and live as if we already are abundant, everything is possible. Nothing is kept from us. It is only our thoughts, old beliefs, and feelings of lack that keep all good things from pouring into our experience. If we *feel* lack, the universe says, "yes, here is more lack for you." When we *feel* abundant, the universe says, "yes, more of that coming right up!"

A TRUE STORY

In the summer of 2003, I was thinking about becoming a Feng Shui practitioner.

For many years, I had been privately studying the ancient art on my own. I had several shelves filled with Feng Shui books. But with every new book I read, my interest only expanded. The more I learned, the more I wanted to know. What I knew, I put to use in my house and my life. I experienced many benefits from my efforts, but often I had questions that went unanswered.

I also developed a strong urge to offer Feng Shui advice to others. If a friend complained of a problem, I knew a Feng Shui cure or remedy that would help. I could match up their personal issues with areas of their home that were cluttered, in disrepair, or possibly missing. When I walked into a house or business, I knew what areas of life were working out well for them and what wasn't working at all.

Feng Shui was an active hobby of mine, but I considered taking it to another level. The idea of becoming qualified to dish out my advice became increasingly attractive. It also seemed like the responsible thing to do.

To become a practitioner, I found, required not only a hefty financial requirement, but also a significant time commitment. I wasn't sure if I could spare either.

There were classes starting in the fall of that year. I debated with myself if I should sign up for them. It was a big commitment. Did I really want to take this on? Would the classes become a burden financially? What about the huge blocks of time required? Did I really want to go back to *school*?

Oh, but what fun it could be! All my questions would get answered. Surely, I could juggle the finances and my time.

My list of pros and cons was of equal size. I went round and round but could not decide. So, I walked on it.

I started out walking and I immediately felt great. It was a gorgeous morning. A true and perfect summer day. I was aware of the fullness and abundance of life that was all around me. The trees were still lush and green. The sky was a lapis blue, with not a cloud in sight. I could hear a flock of starlings chattering busily among themselves. As I approached them, hundreds of birds took off before me. The loud racket they made sounded like a symphony. An abundance of birds and sound.

A little while later, I saw a hawk's feather—large, impressive, and in perfect condition. It was directly in my path. I looked up and saw a red-tailed hawk soaring in the sky above me. The feather was a gift. Time stood still for a moment. I watched how his majestic flight appeared to be so effortless. Suddenly, caught in the present moment, a concern about my own future time felt almost ridiculous.

I pulled myself out of my reverie and continued on. To my complete surprise, I saw a dollar bill lying on the side of the path. I picked it up and saw another, then another. After a few more steps, there was another one. Seven in all. Seven, the mystical, spiritual number. Where did these scattered dollar bills come from? I was on a remote path in the woods! It seemed incredible that someone could have dropped seven bills and not taken notice.

The answer to my question was quite clear. Do it. I would have abundance of both time and money.

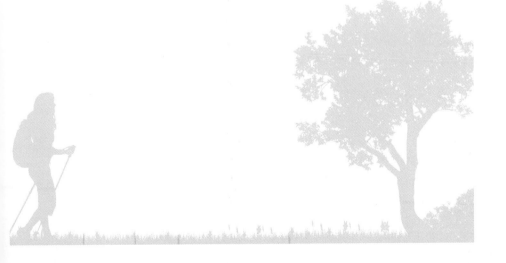

~ GAME EIGHT ~
THE "WALK AWAY" GAME

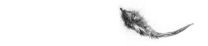

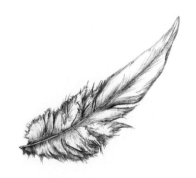

DON'T GO HOME UNTIL
YOU FEEL BETTER.

I stroll along serenely, with my eyes, my shoes, my rage, forgetting everything.
—Pablo Neruda

TIME: 30 MINUTES OR MORE

WHEN TO PLAY:

- You want to change a limiting belief.
- You need inspiration.
- You have been ill.
- You are fighting with someone.
- You want to break a habit.
- You are worried or anxious.

- You are feeling stuck.
- You want to lose weight.
- You feel like your life is out of control.
- You are feeling sorry for yourself.
- You want to end a relationship.
- You are repeating unproductive life patterns.
- You are procrastinating.

HOW TO PLAY:

Take a few long, deep breaths and state your intention. Begin walking at a comfortable pace. During the first several minutes, think about what has been bothering you or about something you want to change.

When you feel ready, make a clear decision to leave it in the past and walk away from it. Keep moving forward. Choose to leave "it" behind you. Announce out loud, "I am leaving _____ behind me. I am walking away now." Repeat this phrase over and over as a mantra. You can use a visualization, perhaps imagining that you are dropping a heavy suitcase and walking away from it. Feel your body getting lighter as you continue to walk farther and farther away from the past. You are looking ahead and moving forward.

After about five minutes, stop walking and speaking. While facing forward, begin to walk backward. Continue for at least twenty to thirty steps. Notice how awkward your body feels to be moving in this way. Feel how it throws off your sense of direction and balance. You cannot see where you are going because you are looking at where you've been! This is exactly what living in the past does to the momentum of your daily life.

Begin to walk forward again, acknowledging and announcing "I am leaving _____ behind me. I am walking forward now." Visualize yourself moving away from what you do not want in your life. See yourself letting it stay behind you, and know you are moving into your future. After approximately five minutes, stop and walk backward again for twenty to thirty steps. Feel the discomfort. Let yourself realize how walking backward breaks your momentum.

Repeat the sequence at least two more times.

The game should last at least thirty minutes. Every five minutes or so, stop and walk backward twenty to thirty steps. You should walk backward at least four times during the walk.

The game is simple, but effective. It has a way of jarring you into the present moment. During the game, you physically move your body backward. This symbolically represents what it is like to be constantly thinking about the past. If you are repeating unproductive habits, procrastinating, or acting out patterns of old, worn-out beliefs, you are not moving forward in life. They keep you off balance and stuck in the past. You may be facing the right direction, but you are not going forward. The past pulls you backward. This game will help you recognize, on a physical, mental, and spiritual level, what happens to you, and ultimately to your life, when you continue to revisit the past.

Letting go of past situations, memories, conversations, and old habits will free up energy and momentum for the future. Breaking habits and patterns that no longer serve you will move you forward in your life with clarity and balance.

~ THE SOUL SCOOP ~

EARTHING

When was the last time you sat under your favorite tree or walked in the grass barefooted? Do you even think about it? Our fast-paced lives drive us forward with shoes on our feet and a phone in our hand. Walking outside while barefooted is often reserved for a once-a-year beach vacation. In a very real way, we have lost our connection to the ground beneath our feet, to the Earth that supports us.

The simple practice of reconnecting with the Earth's energy field is called Earthing.

Earthing, also referred to as grounding, is a method of restoring balance to the energy field in our body by connecting with the energy field in the Earth. Mother Earth is continuously offering up a generous supply of energy. Think of the body as a depleted battery, and the Earth is the recharger. We can recharge, or get grounded, by having direct bodily contact with the Earth. Actually touching the Earth is a behavior that has gone missing with our current lifestyle.

To practice Earthing and get grounded, we can sit or lie directly on the ground. We can take a walk outside barefooted or sit in a chair and let our bare feet touch the ground. According to the Earthing experts, thirty to forty minutes is the preferable time, but shorter periods, with more frequency, will work too. Earthing is safe, natural, and free for all to use.

If you incorporate Earthing into your life, you can reap many more benefits than just getting an energy charge. Earthing can also calm you and lift that frazzled feeling that comes with being overwhelmed. It balances our bioelectrical systems, which results in physiological benefits such as reducing pain and inflammation. Earthing can help you reduce stress by lowering cortisol levels. It may help you sleep better. Earthing can reduce your blood pressure, prevent aging, ease anxiety and depression, and eliminate jet lag.

A doctor friend of mine practices Earthing by gardening in his bare feet. I walk around outside barefooted as much as possible. In spring and summer, I like to sit and drink my morning coffee on my back porch steps, with my feet firmly planted in the grass. If I am working on my computer for several hours and start to feel a little foggy, all I have to do is go outside without shoes and walk around my yard for a few minutes. I will be refreshed and restored.

Recently, I took a step too quickly and twisted my ankle. I went outside, took off my shoes, and sat with both feet connected to the Earth. In about five minutes, all the pain subsided. My ankle never swelled. I was back up and in fine shape in ten minutes.

Experiment for yourself. The next time you stub your toe or bang your elbow, go outside and ground yourself for ten minutes to reduce the pain and inflammation. Use Earthing to promote a sense of well-being or to increase vitality. Practice Earthing for a few minutes before you soul step. Do the breathing, and set your intention in your bare feet and then slip on your shoes and go.

~ GAME NINE ~
CHANGE YOUR STORY

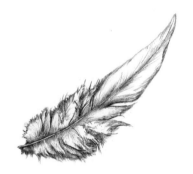

TELL A DIFFERENT STORY AND LIVE A DIFFERENT RESULT.

On the path that leads to nowhere I have sometimes found my soul!
—Corine Roosevelt Robinson

TIME: 30 MINUTES OR MORE

WHEN TO PLAY:

- You feel like a victim.
- You have been ill.
- You are repeating negative patterns in your life.
- You are sad or depressed.
- You are worried or anxious.
- You are feeling stuck.

- You are experiencing unfortunate circumstances.
- You have negative self-talk.
- You feel unloved or unworthy.
- You are lonely.
- You need fresh ideas.
- You want to manifest a desired outcome.
- You feel guilty.

HOW TO PLAY:

Take a few long, deep breaths and state your intention. Begin walking at a comfortable pace. Allow your thoughts to drift naturally to the circumstances of your life. How do you feel about your life in general? Are you currently satisfied? Are you happy? If not, why not? What has been bothering you? What are your complaints? Tell yourself your story. Be honest with yourself and say exactly how you are feeling. Let yourself go. Tell it like it is, or how you feel that it is.

Listen, really listen, to yourself. Pay attention to the words and general tone that you use. You may need to talk out loud to stay focused. Listening to how you talk to yourself and being able to hear the story you tell yourself is the most important aspect at the beginning of this game.

Notice how you are feeling. See how your thoughts and your words create negative- or positive-feeling emotions. Especially listen to the negativity. Watch for repeated phrases or themes.

Break your story down into individual sentences and really hear exactly what you have been saying to yourself. When you allow yourself to examine specific statements, you may realize that much of what you tell yourself is false. Often our thoughts are reactionary and habitual. They may not necessarily be true.

Do you automatically believe everything you think? Should you? Is it the absolute truth? Try to bring yourself to an understanding that your thoughts are simply thoughts. You can control them. You can choose to believe them or choose to change them. Much of our self-talk is habitual and goes unnoticed and unchallenged. Often, we blindly believe everything we think.

When you have exhausted the tale of your life or the specific situation you are in, stop; take a pause and a few slow, deep breaths.

Begin walking again, but this time deliberately tell a different story. Reframe your dialogue in a more positive way. Create a new version for yourself and only use positive and uplifting words. As you continue to walk, you should move into even more powerful statements. The idea is to gradually change the words until you have a fabulous, new version of your story. You can focus on the tale at large or choose a particular sentence or two that has created a theme in your life.

You want to finish the game with a new story that you want to actually live.

For example, in your original version you might have said, "Nothing ever goes right for me." Your narrative continued on, but this line in particular is repeated. It is your theme song. It feels like a life pattern for you. Most of the negative situations in your life seem to eventually boil down to this line, that nothing ever goes right for you.

A newer, more gentle and truer version would be "Sometimes things do go right for me." You can reflect on this and list a few things. "I woke up this morning in good health." "I have employment that supports me." "I love the neighborhood where I live." "I found a convenient parking space at the market when I was in a hurry this morning." It is a fact that some things *do* go right for you.

You will want to then challenge the validity of the first version. It is simply not true that *nothing* ever goes right for you. When you really start to think about it, the statement is absurd. With this realization, you can reach for more empowering and truthful statements. A declaration that feels truer now may be "Many things actually do go right for me." And you can now believe it, because you can name a few things that have in the past gone right for you.

As you continue walking, begin to tell the new and improved story that you want to live. In this example, you would make statements such as "Everything goes right for me" and "I am always at the right place at the right time."

At first, the new spin on the old story might feel awkward, even uncomfortable. Notice how you feel as you reach for creative ways to retell your story. Be attentive to how different words create different emotions. How you have been framing the experience of your life in your thoughts is very important. In a very real way, your self-talk creates the circumstances of your life. What you think determines how you feel. How you feel attracts what you experience.

Be watchful of words such as "never" and "always." These words are dooming, disempowering, and most likely false. There is no way out of "never" and "always."

This is a most powerful game. Played repeatedly, it will completely transform how you think. It will change your self-talk, and your self-talk will change what shows up for you in life.

~ THE SOUL SCOOP ~

LAW OF ATTRACTION

Many people are familiar with the idea of the law of attraction. The law of attraction casts a very wide net that is full of ideas and information. It carries the promise that we can change our reality and "get what we want." It tells us that "like attracts like" and that thoughts are real and measurable things. If we can think positive thoughts, we can create positive experiences. We know that if we put our mind to it, it is possible to manipulate outcomes with intention. We can imagine things into being. The entire concept of the law of attraction is exquisite and daunting simultaneously.

So why do so many of us have trouble getting the results that we want?

This question turns the attention from universal energy principles straight to our own subconscious mind. Like a computer hard drive, our subconscious mind holds all the old programming fed to us as children. It operates without judgment and, in many ways, controls us. It acts as our default program, and it kicks in the minute we let our guard down.

Its purpose is to serve us, like the captain of the ship, and it is basically there to help us. For instance, we do not have to relearn how to drive a car every time we want to go somewhere. Our subconscious mind has stored that program for us. Without even thinking about it, we can jump in the car and go.

However, the subconscious mind also holds deep, core beliefs that we have accumulated along the way. Some of our beliefs, or programs, might not serve us very well and can sabotage us when we try to create the life we want. Underlying our best efforts is a belief system that sticks to us like glue. Our programming is unique to us, depending on what we experienced as children. The beliefs that we are not good enough, that we don't deserve happiness, that we are unlovable, and that there isn't enough to go around are a few of the common themes that can play in the background of our lives and keep us stuck.

After we have exhausted all the tricks of the trade, and not much in our lives has changed, we need to examine our core beliefs.

Our beliefs, which are thoughts that we consciously or unconsciously think over and over again, eventually create the story that is our life. If deep down you think that money is the root of all evil, don't expect to increase your financial status anytime soon. You may want more money, or a better job, or a fat savings account, but your underlying and dominant programming will sabotage your efforts. The captain of your ship is protecting you from the evils of money.

We will attract to us what we ultimately believe, even if it is not what we are wanting. This, in turn, produces life situations that prove to us what we already think. Our life reinforces our core beliefs. It is the law of attraction in action. We can point to the evidence in our experiences and say, "See, it's true." The universe bends over backward to make us right.

To change an undesirable or false belief, we first need to identify what programs are running us. Then we can trace their history, challenge their validity, and begin to change them.

It all begins with our basic beliefs, which dominate how and what we think. Our thoughts determine how we feel. How we think and what we feel become the story of our lives. We are vibrational beings. We live in a vibrational environment. Our thoughts and feelings are made up of vibrations. Our feelings, or our emotions, are the powerful creative signals that we emit out into the universal energy field. Our emotional vibrations sent out into the universe are what will draw to us similar circumstances that match. Like attracts like. It is our emotions that do the creating.

Think of your emotions as powerful creative magnets. We attract circumstances, people, and things (or lack of things) to match the vibrations of our emotions. Simply put, we will get more of what we feel. If we dominantly feel depressed, angry, or sorry for ourselves, that is the vibe we are emanating out into the universal energy field. The universal field is like a mirror. It will reflect back what appears before it. We get back what we give out.

The universe only knows one language, and that is the language of vibrations. In order to change our lives and get what we want, we need to communicate to the universe in the only language that it knows. We are doing it all the time anyway with our emotions. We need to be conscious of the way we feel. We need to deliberately be aware of what emotional signals we send out, because that's what we will get more of in the days ahead.

The universe is benevolent and generous. Its language is vibration, but it only has one answer to everything and that answer is yes. Are you angry most of the time? The universe says, "Yes, okay, I will give you more reasons to feel angry." Do you feel like a victim, feeling powerless in many areas of your life? The universe will always agree with you. It says, "Yes, you are powerless, and let me prove it to you." The universe responds to you, not the other way around.

When it comes to the emotions, I like to offer this advice: "Feel what you feel; just don't stay there too long." This means that there is no need to fear or deny our feelings. We are human, after all, and have a marvelous capacity to experience a wide range of emotions. There is no benefit in trying to ignore or press down our emotions. Give yourself permission to feel your frustration or envy or anger. Feel it, process it, and then let it go. The sooner the better.

Your emotions are the powerful creative force that will change your life. Find ways to make yourself consistently feel better. Examine what you really say to yourself. Become aware of the negative messages you feed yourself that keep you stuck in negative emotions. Disrupting your core beliefs by allowing yourself to root them out and challenge them will change the way you feel. And the way you feel determines what you attract.

～ GAME TEN ～
TIME TO RHYME

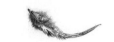

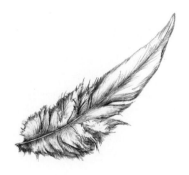

CREATE A RHYME TO EASE YOUR WOES, AND WATCH HOW EASILY LIFE BEGINS TO FLOW.

I can feel my soul dance, walking in rhyme.
—Chante Moore

TIME: 30 MINUTES OR MORE

WHEN TO PLAY:

- You feel tired or fatigued.
- You are having trouble sleeping.
- You feel like a victim.
- You have a negative attitude.
- You have been ill.

- You are repeating negative patterns in your life.
- You are depressed, worried, or anxious.
- You are feeling stuck.
- You are unhappy.
- You have negative self-talk.
- You feel unloved or unworthy.
- You want to change something in your life.
- You want to manifest a desired outcome.

HOW TO PLAY:

Before you begin, choose a rhyme that applies to your situation. Your rhyme should be upbeat and positive. The words should redirect a negative thought or situation that you are experiencing. Phrase your rhyme in the present tense. Keep the focus of the words on what you wish to create for yourself.

To begin, take a few long, deep breaths and state your intention. Start out walking at a comfortable pace. Say the rhyme that you have chosen. Repeat it over and over. Listen to the words you are saying. Staying very present, allow yourself to feel every word of the rhyme. Unlike the "Affirmation Walk," your rhyming should not become just sounds you are making. You should give attention to each and every word that is being said. You should step in time to the rhythm of your words. In this way you are using your body to put emphasis on the words.

You can repeat your rhymes silently or out loud. Saying the rhyme out loud helps your attention stay on the words. Sound is healing to the body. Allow your voice to resonate through your entire being.

You can play with the tone, beat, and volume of your words.

Continue rhyming the entire walk without breaking your stride or the rhythm of your words.

You will return from the game with a refreshed attitude, a revived body, and a nourished spirit.

A fun and creative twist on the game is to make up the rhymes as you are walking. You can choose one line and use this line as your starting point. When you get stuck coming up with new rhymes, return to the first sentence and begin again. Your soul will offer relevant rhymes as you walk, if you walk in a relaxed, nonresistant way.

For example, you can begin with the statement "Life loves me." Continue using that sentence as your starting point. "Life loves me and I am free. All good things come to me easily. I am so very healthy because life loves me." You can return to the first line as often as you need to, as new rhymes occur to you. This should flow evenly, without long thinking gaps in between rhymes. Should you get stuck, return to the first sentence. In this case, "Life loves me." Repeat the first line until a new rhyme comes to you. You will be amazed at how easy it is to continue to come up with new rhymes.

As you go through the day, you may find yourself repeating rhymes you used during your walk. Your rhymes can be used as affirmations. Using affirmations in a rhyming way helps them sink into our subconscious minds. Our minds remember them. Repetition of a rhyme is a valuable way to change old programming buried deep in our subconscious mind.

My niece, Sara, devised a clever way to diffuse sibling rivalry between her children. She came up with a few rhymes to say when things start getting out of hand. She says them first, and the kids repeat them. "It's okay. It's all right. There's no need to start a fight" and "All is well. Can't you tell?" These simple lines have become a way to change the point of attention and restore peace in the home.

Rhyming is a playful way to redirect our thoughts and reprogram our subconscious mind. It can connect us to our inner child. It is an easy and effective method to replace old programming with new ways of thinking and being.

You will find examples of rhymes in chapter 6.

A TRUE STORY

Years ago, my friend Gina told me the story of how her elderly next-door neighbor helped change her life.

Gina was a single mother, had full-time employment, and was also a student working on her master's degree. Her life was overloaded and hectic. She was busy, overwhelmed, and often frantic. It seemed as if she was always rushing off in a hurry. She left her house early in the morning and came home late at night.

She was friendly with the old woman who lived next door, but hadn't had the time to really nurture a relationship. Gina saw her sitting at her window every morning when she left her house. They would smile and wave to each other.

Every day, the old woman watched Gina running out the door in a chaotic way. Along with her purse, her bags, and her child, she carried folders that bulged with papers. More often than not, she would drop something while digging in her purse for her keys. Her life was disorganized, and many times she would realize that her keys were still inside. Several times she had locked herself out and had to climb through the side window of her house. For many months, the old woman watched it all.

One day, Gina left her home later than usual. She saw the woman sitting on her small porch. The woman waved for her to come over. Gina did not have the time for a conversation, but out of politeness, she went. The woman didn't want a conversation. She didn't lecture her with the wisdom of her life. She simply said, "Say this when you feel stressed or fearful," and then she told her a rhyme.

I am the place where God shines through.

And if I be relaxed and free,

He'll carry out his work through me.

When she got into her car, she scribbled it down. As she moved into the rest of her day, Gina repeated the rhyme over and over so she wouldn't forget it. It was simple, but she could not deny that it was profound.

Many years later, she told me how those words were just the message that she needed to hear that day.

She said that the rhyme became her affirmation and literally changed her life. It brought peace and calmness to her when she said it. Conditions soon smoothed out and life got easier. She effortlessly got more organized, went on to get her PhD, and soon after married a wonderful man. One could say she is living happily ever after.

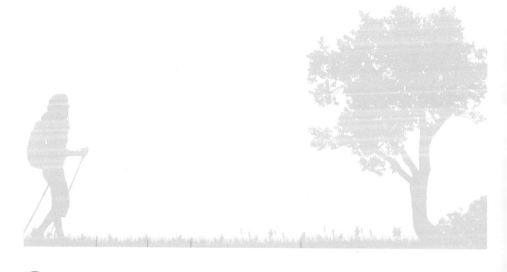

~ CHAPTER SIX ~
WALK YOUR TALK

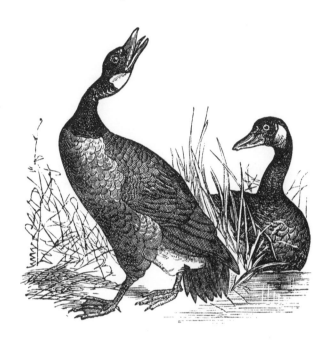

A REFERENCE LIST OF AFFIRMATIONS AND RHYMES.

I have arrived. I am home. In the here. In the now.
I am solid. I am free. In the ultimate I dwell.
—Thich Nhat Hanh

In the 1990s, my obsession with New Thought authors led me to the writings of Florence Scovel Shinn. It was in her books that I was first introduced to the idea of using rhyme and affirmations to change an unwanted situation in my life. Originally an illustrator of books, Shinn became a true pioneer and a leading author in the New Thought movement. In the nineteenth century and on through to the early twentieth century, New Thought speakers and authors blazed the trail for the more modern New Age era that came later.

My interest soon led me to find affirmation icon Louise Hay. Author and founder of her own publishing company, she, too, became a pioneer and giant in the field. She first proved, and then told the world, that our thoughts and our words can change our lives.

It would be a challenge to read, write, hear, or say an affirmation without realizing the influence of Florence Scovel Shinn or Louise Hay. Important to remember, however, is that the most powerful affirmations and rhymes are the ones you create yourself. The biggest and best results will be had with words that are tailored for your specific situation.

Affirmations are positive words that are said over and over to create a change in your thinking. They can be used to turn around and replace negative thoughts that you repeatedly tell yourself. For instance, if you think that "there isn't enough time in a day," you can begin to replace those words with "everything is done in perfect timing."

The shorter the affirmation, the easier it is to remember and incorporate into your life. Rhymes should be simple and consist of one or two lines. They should be lighthearted and fun to say. When creating your own affirmations or rhymes, use empowering and positive words. Phrase your affirmation or rhyme as if it is already true and you are stating a fact. Use words such as "now" and "attract." The words "I am" are the most powerful and creative words you can use to begin any sentence.

The affirmations and rhymes below are divided into subject sections, but they are not limited for use in just that way. The subjects simply serve as a guide.

AFFIRMATIONS

ABUNDANCE

All good comes to me.
As I thank, I receive.
Everything I need comes to me in the most divine and perfect way.
I am abundant. The universe is generous and never fails me.
I am grateful for my abundance. Life is good to me.
I am open to receive.
I am prosperous. I live my life in abundance.
I attract to me only good. I attract to me everything I need.
I have everything I need, when I need it.
I see abundance everywhere I go.
Money comes to me easily and effortlessly.
Money flows naturally into my life.
Nature is abundant. Life is abundant. I am abundant.
Thank you. Thank you. Thank you.
What is mine comes to me.

HEALTH

I am grateful for my body. I am grateful for my health.
I have perfect health. I am protected. I am safe.
I am strong. I am healthy. I am perfect.
I am surrounded with a loving perfection. All is well.
I am whole. I am perfect. I am well.
I attract what is good for me. All is well. I am well.
I can relax now. My body knows what to do.
I love myself. I am perfect in every way.
I now bring balance to my body, to my mind, to my soul.
I surround myself with the white light of the Christ consciousness.
I walk through life in perfect harmony. Only good comes to me.
My perfect body knows what to do. I am perfect health.
My body is in balance. My mind is in balance. My spirit is in balance.
Nothing has gone wrong. Everything is right. I am perfection.
When I listen to my body, I know what to do.

RELATIONSHIPS

I accept myself. I love myself.
I accept everyone just as they are.
I am you. You are me. We are one.
I am surrounded with love. Love is all I see.
I attract the perfect partner.
I forgive myself. I forgive others. I go free.
I give love. I am open to receive love. Everything is perfect.
I love you. I am sorry. Please forgive me. Thank you.
I now open myself to give only love. I now open myself to receive only love.
I radiate love. I attract only love.
My heart is open to receive love.
The right people show up for me at the right time.
Only love comes into my experience.
Perfect people. Perfect timing. Perfect love.
What I see in you, I am.

WELL-BEING

All is well. All is always well.
Everything is unfolding for my highest and greatest good.
I accept all that I am. I am whole and perfect.
I am always at the right place at the right time.
I am being guided. I listen to my heart.
I am safe. I am harmony. I am love.
I breathe in love. I breathe out fear.
I love life and life loves me.
I now release what no longer serves me. I let go effortlessly.
I surround myself with white light. I am safe.
I trust myself. I follow my highest good.
Life is always good to me.
Nothing has gone wrong. I am always in the universal flow.
My highest self knows what to do.
My mind is clear. I am focused. I am present.

RHYMES

ABUNDANCE

Abundance is everything I see.
Abundance is a part of me.

All good comes to me,
easily and continuously.

All good things come my way.
All good things are here to stay.

Everything I need comes to me.
I attract money easily.

I am happy. I am free.
Money is just energy.

I relax. I am free.
Abundance is natural to me.

I receive all that I need.
I relax and let God lead.

I trust myself and I am free.
All good things come to me.

Money, money everywhere.
I have plenty and I can share.

Wealth is mine and here to stay.
I have wealth in every way.

HEALTH

All this day I am complete,
by blessing everything I eat.

Good health is mine on this day.
Good health is mine and here to stay.

I am strong in every way.
I am whole and perfect every day.

I am well this whole day through.
Only my perfect health is true.

I bless my body and I go free.
My body is the perfect me.

I hand myself over to God above.
He fills me up with only love.

I listen to my body and eat what I should.
Everything I eat is for my good.

My body is perfect in every way.
My body is healthy every day.

My health is my wealth.

Perfect health flows through me.
Perfect health is all I see.

RELATIONSHIPS

All is right. All is well.
In perfect love is where I dwell.

I am happy. I am free.
The perfect people come to me.

I give love on this day,
and love shows up in every way.

I let things go. I let things roll.
It keeps me free. It keeps me whole.

I love you and you love me.
We live our life in harmony.

I accept perfect love for me.
Perfect love is all I see.

It's okay. It's all right.
There's no need to start a fight.

These three I attract easily.
Happiness, love, and harmony.

This I know is true.
I love me and I love you.

When I relax, love comes my way.
When I let go, it comes to stay.

WELL-BEING

All good things come to me.
I live my life in harmony.

All is well on this day.
It is perfect in every way.

All of my actions are inspired and true.
I move about perfectly with all that I do.

Everything I do
is divine and true.

Everything I need to know is revealed to me.
Everything I need to do is done effortlessly.

Everything I need to know is revealed to me.
I relax. I am free.

I am happy. I am free.
Only good comes to me.

I am surrounded by white light.
It protects me day and night.

I am the place where God shines through.
And if I be relaxed and free,
He'll carry out his work through me.

I love myself. I am free.
Only good comes to me.

CHAPTER SEVEN

STEPPING OUT, STEPPING IN

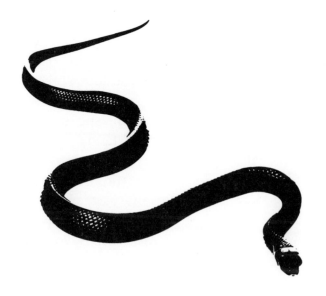

A LIST OF SIGNS AND OMENS.

The bird that cries korokoro *in the rice field I know to be a* hototogisu—*yet it may have been my father; it may have been my mother.*
—Zen saying

Nature teaches us everything we need to know. It will answer all of our questions. It will always tell us the truth.

If we are willing to interact with the natural world, we can develop a personal and intimate relationship with nature. When we are open to communication, demonstrate respect, and offer gratitude, our relationship with nature will deepen with time and can become a true partnership.

Nature collaborates with us when we soul step. It will provide unlimited information in the form of signs and omens, but it is up to us to interpret it. When we put forth a genuine effort to connect, the easier it becomes to understand the messages that nature gives. The more you trust, the greater your rewards.

How do we know if something we encounter is a sign or omen? A specific sign or omen will come in a startling or unusual way. It will grab your attention and be impossible to ignore. Often, it will cause you to pause or stop what you are doing. It might be amazing and inspire a sense of awe. But it is important to note that everything, every single thing, we experience in nature can be interpreted. The subtle breeze, the flock of birds, and the single wildflower all are communication from nature. As you begin to recognize and interpret the fantastic messages, the subtle language of nature becomes easier to understand.

The guide below will help you interpret the signs and omens you receive while soul stepping. The interpretations are intended to point you in the right direction. They are meant to act as prompts for you to discover your deeper meanings. Allow them to inspire higher soul insights that relate to you personally. Always trust your own intuition.

~ A ~

ACCIDENT

To witness an accident of any type may be telling you that someone is
  being wrongfully blamed.
Are you blaming yourself for something?
This may be the time to release guilt.
This may be a reminder that there are always two sides to every story.

ACORN

An acorn can represent hope.
Finding an acorn can be the promising start of something that will grow
  substantially larger.
This can mean a financial payoff or debts being satisfied.
An acorn can represent the need to begin to save for the future.
It can mean a humble beginning.
It might mean a baby on the way.

AIRPLANE

To see an airplane can mean you will rise above a current issue or state
  of affairs.
It can mean travel or going places, symbolically or literally.
An airplane may mean you need to look to a higher power for guidance
  or assistance.

ANTS

Ants usually indicate work or work issues.
They can be symbolic of a need to work together.
Community effort or cooperation of some kind may be required if you
  see ants.
Ants can also refer to carrying a heavy burden.
Have you been working too hard or carrying more than your share of
  the load?

APPLE

An apple can represent your life force or new beginnings.
You may need nourishment, literally or symbolically.
It may also mean a temptation that is not in your best interest.
An apple may indicate a teacher or a lesson coming into your life.

~ B ~

BABY

A baby may indicate news of a pregnancy.
Babies also represent innocence or new life.
Seeing a baby may bring a new beginning or tell of the birth of a new
    project or undertaking.
You may be given another chance.

BALLOON

To see a balloon in the sky means your hopes will be fulfilled. Make
    a wish.
If it is caught in a tree or otherwise stuck, it can mean there will be effort
    required before your dreams can come true.
Hopes deflated, if you see a balloon on the ground.

BAT

Bats can bring a warning to listen carefully.
They indicate a need to tune into your intuition and follow your instincts.
They may be indicators of change, transformation, or a crossing over
    to the spiritual realm.
Bats can also bring messages from spirit.

BEE

Bees will indicate work or work issues.

They may be telling you to work for the greater good of all.

Bees can also represent a tendency toward selfishness on your part, or on the part of another.

Or they may indicate that you are giving too much to others and compromising your own needs.

There may be a need to see the bigger picture.

BEETLE

A beetle can indicate longevity.

Seeing a beetle may be telling you to toughen up or that you need to develop a thicker skin.

A beetle can act as a totem of protection.

BIRD

Any bird is a divine creature and a messenger from heaven.

Pay attention to the specific type of bird and what it is doing.

Birds bring joy, but they can also warn you to be cautious.

Spirits often take the form of birds.

BLUE JAY

A blue jay is a symbol of boldness and courage.

These birds can represent a tendency toward bullying or vanity.

They are great mimics, so stay authentic and true to your own voice.

A blue jay can indicate gossip.

Pay attention to the words you have been speaking. Be kind and use your voice to uplift others.

BREEZE

A soft, whispering breeze can be a sign of spirit. It can confirm that your soul is working with you.

A light breeze can mean you are on the right path.

If you are looking for a yes or no answer, a sudden soft breeze will likely mean a yes.

BRIDGE

A bridge can mean a connection to be made.
It may indicate a time period before an opportunity manifests.
It may be telling you there is a way to get over something.
What do you need to bridge in your life?
You may need to take time off or change the subject to have a breakthrough of any kind.
A bridge can indicate a between time, neither here nor there.
Is there a decision to be made?

BUTTERFLY

A butterfly is a symbol of freedom.
It can mean a change for the better.
Butterflies also represent metamorphosis and transformation.
A butterfly may be telling you to bring levity to a situation.
If there are two, they can be a wonderful relationship totem, signifying happiness.

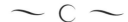 C

CAT

Cats bring mysterious and magical solutions.
Cats are a symbol of silence. Seeing a cat may be a call to meditate or find space for quiet reflection.
They may be a sign to talk less, listen more.
There may be a need to establish independence or cultivate patience.
Do you need to bring balance to an area of your life?
Cats are watchers. Pay attention.

CEMETERY

A cemetery can mean it is time to honor or forgive loved ones who have passed.

It may be a call to explore your past or your ancestors.
Feeling drawn to walk through a cemetery can indicate there will be messages from spirit.

CHILDREN

When seeing children, it should be noted what they are doing. Are they playing and laughing? Are they fighting or sitting alone quietly? Their behavior will indicate the meaning of the sign.
Happy children can bring joy or a bright outcome.
Children fighting or being disagreeable means caution or a need to examine your own behavior.
Children may indicate a level of immaturity in you or someone else.
Seeing children may be a call to connect with your childhood or your inner child.
There may be a need to take more time to play.

CLOUDS

Dark clouds can mean obstacles or caution.
White, puffy clouds can mean hope.
Can you distinguish any shapes or symbols in the formation of the clouds?
Pay attention to the movement of the clouds and the speed of the movement.
Or are they not moving at all?

COIN

Finding a coin is a sign of abundance.
Money or luck is coming.
The larger the denomination, the larger the luck or sum.

CROW

Crows will always bring a message.
They are extremely intelligent and vocal.

Are you using your own intelligence or making emotional choices?
Do you need to speak up or use your voice in some way?
Pay attention to the number of crows.
One for sorrow, two for joy.
Three for a girl, four for a boy.
Five for silver, six for gold.
Seven for a secret that's never been told.

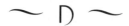

DAFFODILS

Daffodils are an omen of hope.
They represent a new beginning or another chance.
Daffodils may indicate that the time to act on something is now.

DEER

Deer are symbols of gentleness.
Kindness may be required.
They can represent a need to tread softly or to slow down.
When seeing deer, stop and listen to your own heart.
They may indicate a need to listen more closely and hear what isn't being
    said.
They can be a symbol or totem for mother.

DOG

Dogs can represent friends or associates.
They indicate loyalty or the need to trust. But they will also tell you who
    should not be trusted.
They will act as mirrors to your own true self.
They are protectors and guardians.
Pay attention to the specific type of dog, its demeanor, and what it is
    doing.

DRAGONFLY

Dragonflies may mean emotional changes for the better.
They can indicate the need to lighten up or to have some fun.
They are connectors to the spirit and faerie realms.
They can lead you into magical thinking and problem solving.

DUCK

Ducks symbolize that your emotions are involved.
You may need to let an emotional situation roll off your back.
They mean resilience.
You may need to use water in some way as a healing remedy.
Keep yourself hydrated.

~ E ~

EGRET

These elegant birds may be telling you it is time to process your emotions.
It may be time to release negative emotions that you have been holding
    on to for a long time.

ENVELOPE

An envelope means there are messages coming or news is arriving.
Perhaps you need to deliver a message.
An envelope might indicate the need to carefully rehearse your words
    before you speak.

~ F ~

FEATHER

A feather is a gift from nature.

It is usually a positive confirmation.
If you are looking for a yes or no answer, a feather will likely mean a yes.
It can mean your wishes will be fulfilled.

FIRE

Fire is generally a sign of transformation.
A change or release is needed.
Fire may indicate issues with anger.
It can mean that intense emotions need to be processed and resolved.

FISH

Fish are omens of emotions.
There may be a situation in which you feel as if you are drowning.
Go deep inside. Meditate.
Emotions will pass. You will know what to do.
They can also reflect issues with money.
Fish are a sign of abundance.

FLY

A fly can indicate a possible ending.
There may be a need to listen more attentively.
Don't believe everything you hear.
Use discernment with friends and associates.

FOOD

Food may mean you need physical, mental, or spiritual nourishment.
It may mean there is some type of overindulgence.
Self-love is needed.

FORK IN THE ROAD

Coming to a fork in the road always indicates a decision to be made.
You may be struggling with indecision, and it is time to make a choice.

All roads will eventually lead home.
Listen to your heart and soul.

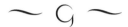

GARBAGE

Garbage means a need to deal with clutter either physically, mentally, or emotionally.
Clean up your act. Get organized.
Garbage is a sign you need to let go of something either literally or symbolically.
Garbage can mean you need to use discernment.

GEESE

Geese are writing totems.
They may mean that flying in a new direction will benefit you.
Geese can lead you into the spiritual and quantum realms.
They can represent your childhood and will help you resolve old issues.
Geese can indicate a need for balance.
They are wonderful relationship totems and mean faithfulness and longevity with a partner.

GOAT

A goat will mean someone is being stubborn.
There may be a need to relax strong opinions and see another viewpoint.
Empathy may be required.
Goats may indicate a need to pay attention to your diet.
They can indicate a healing for digestive or skin issues.

GRAFFITI

Graffiti may be an indicator that you need to express yourself.
Someone may be expressing their feelings inappropriately.

You may be involved in something illicit.
Can you see the writing on the wall?

GRASSHOPPER

Grasshoppers can mean quantum leaps.
They give permission to move forward.
They may indicate that your progress will take a step back but you will
ultimately succeed.
Grasshoppers may show a need to step back and reassess your situation
before plunging ahead.

GROUNDHOG

A groundhog means new opportunities are coming.
A groundhog can bring fresh ideas and indicate new projects being
birthed.
They may indicate a waiting period before you see success.
Keep new ideas and projects to yourself. You may need to wait for the
right time to reveal your ideas.
A groundhog may be telling you it is time to come out and reveal your gifts.
They can indicate something buried from the past that needs to come
to light.

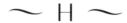

HAWK

Hawks are messengers.
They are protectors.
You may need to pay attention to and trust your inner voice.
Hawks are omens that you are on the right path. Stay your course.
The spirit of a loved one can take the form of a hawk.

HILL

A hill means that there may be more effort required for you to succeed.
There may be obstacles to surmount.
Something in your life may seem hard, but if you persevere, you will
    reach the top.

HORSE

Horses are an omen of strength and freedom.
Horses show how sheer willpower can move you forward.
They mean determination and conviction.
Horses can indicate travel.
They can take you to new heights and provide strength you didn't know
    you had.
They will act as mirrors to your own true self.

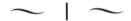

INSECT

Insects can mean a small nuisance.
Are you letting the little things bother you?
Pay attention to the specific type of insect and what it is doing.

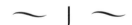

JUMP

Having to jump over anything means you will be able to bypass struggle.
There may be another way to look at a situation.
A problem may be solved in an unconventional way.
It may be time to take a leap of faith.

～ K ～

KEY

A key is a lucky omen.
You will find a way to succeed.
New doors will open for you.
A surprising opportunity may come when you least expect it.
There may be a need for you to unlock something in your life.

KITE

A kite indicates flying high.
It brings hope and success.
It may be necessary to change your course to succeed.

KNIFE

A knife means you should cut ties with someone.
You may need to end a difficult situation.
A knife can mean a fight or argument.
A knife can indicate a dissolved partnership.

～ L ～

LADDER

A ladder can indicate climbing to new heights.
It may mean your current status will rise.
A ladder cautions to take one step at a time.

LADYBUG

A ladybug connects us to our childhood.
It may be time to revive an old interest or connect with someone from the past.

Ladybugs can lead us into the magical faerie realms.
They grant our wishes and give us hope.

LIGHTNING

Lightning is a confirmation of connection with source energy or a higher
     power.
It can bring spirit communication.
Lightning is a sign of a message coming.
Lightning can be a warning.
It is a call to pay attention and stay alert.
Lightning can indicate a flash of genius.

～ M ～

MOLE

Mole can symbolize secrets.
Something unknown may be revealed that will shed light on a current
     situation.
A mole can mean that it is time to let go of little nuisances.
Are you making mountains out of molehills?
What are you being blind to?

MONEY

Money means prosperity and abundance.
It can indicate fruitful investments.
Money gives the green light to advance projects.
It can mean the start-up of a new business.
Money can forecast profits.

MORNING GLORIES

These delicate flowers bring hope and new opportunity.
New ideas or creativity will bloom.

Your desires will come to fruition.
Morning glories may indicate that morning is the best time to act.
You may need to pay attention to timing your actions.

MOTH

Moths indicate change and transformation.
They can bring new relationships.
Moths can indicate news or messages coming in the evening.
Pay attention to your dreams.

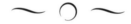

NEST

A nest is a symbol of your home and family.
There may be a need to nurture or be nurtured.
A nest can mean more attention needs to be given to a house or family.
Childhood issues may need to be addressed.
A nest can be a sign of pregnancy or a birth in the family.

OAK TREE

An oak tree is an omen of strength and longevity.
Anything and everything is possible.
An oak tree proves that small effort can produce great rewards.
An oak tree is a call to trust.

PIGEON

Pigeons represent home and family.
They can indicate new relationships.
There may be issues with your house or home.
They can reflect a need to go back home or reconnect with family.
Is there a family member you need to contact?

PINE TREE

A pine tree is an evergreen symbolizing endurance.
It has ties to family.
Pine trees can mean there is emotional healing needed around family issues.
One pine tree can represent mother or father.
These trees can be a sign to let go and surrender to a higher power.

PRAYING MANTIS

A praying mantis brings the message to be patient and wait.
Take time to make decisions. Don't rush into anything.
A praying mantis indicates a need to slow down.
You may need to be still or meditate.

～ R ～

RABBIT

A rabbit is a gentle totem that can mean there will be an abundance of
    opportunity.
It warns us to not make our choices from a place of fear.
A rabbit can be an omen to stop, wait, and lie low until the time is right.
It can indicate a need to go with the flow of life.
A rabbit can increase our psychic abilities.

RAIN

Rain will mean a washing away of what is no longer needed.
It indicates a cleansing and a healing.
Rain can be a symbol of tears or emotional pain.
It can mean a temporary period of strife.
Rain can tell us to use water as a healing modality.

RAINBOW

A rainbow is a promise of better times ahead.
It can mean uplifting news is forthcoming.
It can be an omen of a happy beginning or a happy ending.
A rainbow can be a promise of radiant health or financial abundance.
If you are looking for a yes or no answer, a rainbow will mean a yes.

ROBIN

A robin is a bringer of good news and hope.
It can mean a new beginning or a fresh start.
It represents the season of spring.
Robins carry messages of family and may indicate a need to deal with
    family responsibilities.
A robin may point out a need to spend more time at home.
It may be a sign of a new house or an addition to the family.

ROCKS

Rocks mean stability and endurance against odds.
They are a sign to hold fast and stay true.
They tell us that there is power in quiet strength.
Rocks can mean there is a need to seek out or practice ancient healing
    modalities.

ROSE

A rose is always a blessing.
It can indicate romance or deep and enduring love.
A rose means your prayers will be answered.
It can mean spiritual gifts and financial abundance.
If you are looking for a yes or no answer, a rose will likely mean a yes.

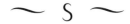

SHELL

A shell is an omen of potential.
It means that all is not lost.
Your answers may not be apparent. They may be hidden right now but
    will be revealed later.
Shells indicate that some time may be required for dreams to come true.

SNAKE

Snakes mean changes and transformation.
They can be guardians and protectors.
They can indicate a need to protect something.
They caution you against shady deals, lies, false friends, and associates.
Snakes can mean money is coming.
Snakes are bringers of the truth.

SPIDER

Spiders are an omen of words and writing.
Pay attention to what is being said, what you read, and what you say.
Say what you mean and mean what you say.
They can warn of getting caught in a trap.

SQUIRREL

A squirrel can be an omen of resourcefulness.
It may indicate a need to shore up resources and plan for the future.
A squirrel can also mean a tendency toward hoarding.
It can help you discern what to keep and what not to keep.

STONES

Stones speak of permanence and what is solid in your life.
They can also mean a short-lived struggle or difficult time.
Stones bring the strength that is required to overcome obstacles.
Stones can be divination tools. Look to see if the stone resembles a
    specific animal or object.
Pay attention to the shape, texture, and color of the stone.

STORM

Storms indicate intensity of emotion.
A sudden storm warns of obstacles ahead.
Storms may indicate heated arguments or a relationship breakup.
Storms are a reminder that there is a higher and greater power at work
    behind the scenes.
A storm can show us how to be humble.

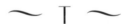

THUNDER

Thunder means pay attention and listen.
It may indicate you are hearing what you want to hear, instead of what
    is actually being said.
It can be a warning to be cautious.
Who has been yelling or shouting?
Thunder can indicate obstacles are ahead, but it also brings the
    promise that they will be temporary.

TOAD

A toad means change, usually for the better.
It is an omen of money coming.
A toad can show up when there are major life changes or during periods of transition.
Toads can help us jump to the next level.
They can assist us with timing and patience.
Toads can help us know when to wait and when to act.
Toad can indicate a visitor.

TOY

A toy can indicate a need to have more fun or be more playful.
Any toy may be a call to connect with your inner child.
Toys may be symbols of childhood issues that you need to address.
Toys may bring up a forgotten memory that will have a relevant and current message.
They can tell us not to take ourselves so seriously.

TREE

Trees symbolize stability, strength, and endurance.
They tell us to stand tall and stand up for ourselves.
They may indicate a need to put down roots.
Trees may be advising us to get grounded.
They represent family.
Is there a family member you need to spend time with or contact?

TUNNEL

A tunnel indicates a journey within.
It can means secrets, either kept or exposed.
A tunnel may mean that a problem or issue lies deep within the subconscious.
They tell us to love the shadow parts of ourselves.
A tunnel can mean you need to bring light to the past in order to move forward.

TURTLE

A turtle indicates a need to take your time or slow down.
Turtles are symbols of longevity.
They can act as protectors.
Is there a need to watch your back?
They can be omens of abundance or long-term investments.
A turtle makes us remember that breath is life. Practice long, slow,
  deep breathing.

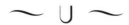

UMBRELLA

An umbrella is an indication that self-care is needed.
Are you always putting other peoples needs before your own?
An umbrella may mean something needs protected.
Keep new ideas under cover until the time is right to reveal them.

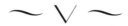

VEHICLES

A vehicle may mean a trip or journey.
It may indicate that a project will soon be off and running.
It may be time to move forward.
Vehicles may symbolize that it is time to leave the past behind and look
  to the future.

VIOLETS

This tiny flower offer the hope of a renewal.
Violets indicate a new beginning and the end of hard times.
They are faerie flowers and can mean that magic is afoot.
They are symbols of forgiveness.

~ W ~

WALL

A wall can indicate obstacles to overcome.
A wall can mean you need to establish personal boundaries.
You may need to protect your time or your assets.
Are you feeling like you are up against a wall?
A wall may mean you need to go in a different direction.

WASP

A wasp can mean there is a need to accept others as they are.
Wasps may mean you need to calm your anger to get better results.
They may indicate a time of cooperating with others.
They can be a call to curb selfishness and look to the greater good of all.
Wasps may warn of words that sting.

WATER

Water can be a symbol of emotions.
It can be a call to bring forth and heal buried emotions.
This may be a time of cleansing, detoxing, or healing.
Water is also a sign of money and abundance.
Water can indicate that new ideas and opportunities are coming.

WIND

The wind blows to indicate change.
The wind can be a sign of spirit.
It may mean a new life force or another chance.
The wind can be a confirmation of soul communication.

WORDS

Words are messages.
Is there any personal or symbolic meaning in the words?
Words may indicate something that needs to be said or written.
Pay attention to the location of the words. Are they on a tall billboard,
    written on a wall, or maybe on a torn paper you see on the ground?

WREN

Wrens are positive signs of hope and joy.
They are symbols of good luck.
They may indicate a time to use your voice to uplift yourself or others.
Wrens bring perseverance and tell us not to give up.
They may indicate a move or a relocation.
Music may be used as a healing modality.

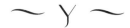

YELLOW JACKET

Yellow jackets are a sign that caution is needed.
Do not aggravate a situation.
They can warn us to think before we speak.
Are you responding or reacting?

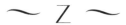

ZINNIA

These flowers can mean that a sense of humor and laughter is needed.
Are you taking yourself too seriously?
They may indicate a need to wear brighter colors.
They are signs of better times to come.

~ CHAPTER EIGHT ~
ANIMAL TOTEMS

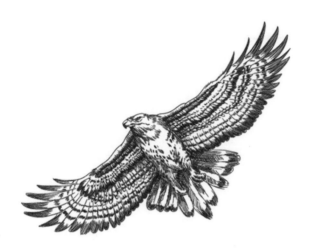

"Who were the sages who taught the Buddha?" the Master was asked.
He replied, "The dog and the cat."
—A Zen Mondo

On this planet, we coexist with nature and with animals. Animals are natural wonders of our world. They are the great teachers for us, if we are willing to learn from them. They give us messages and gifts of spirit. They inspire awe. They bring us joy.

Animals will willingly work with us, if we open ourselves to the messages that they bring. They are guides and can act as a bridge between our physical lives and the spiritual realm. A whole world of possibility and knowledge opens up when you begin to invite, notice, and appreciate the gift of animals.

We are each born with one or two animal totems that will assist us during our entire lifetime. These specific animals act as spirit guides, protectors, and teachers for us. Once you discover what they are, you can be attentive to them and can call on them for help or guidance. You will recognize the importance of the moment when they make an appearance in your life.

Our totems will not always show up in real-life situations, particularly if they are exotic animals. The large cats, such as lions and tigers, may work with us in the form of domesticated cats. Wolves may guide us in the form of dogs. They may show up in dreams. Someone may send us a card or give us a gift with an image of our totem. We may see a documentary or use a business logo with a totem design. Once we know them and acknowledge them, they will repeatedly show up in one way or another. Our lifetime totems often come to assist us during periods of transformation or during major life events.

Our two strongest emotions, love and fear, will often reveal our birth totems. Perhaps as long as you can remember, you have loved dogs or horses, or both. Maybe you are petrified of spiders or snakes or have repetitive nightmares about bears that chase you.

To discover your animal birth totems, you will want to ask yourself what animals do you love or fear. What animals repeatedly show up in your dreams? Was there an animal that you were particularly fond of as child? Did you sleep with or carry a specific stuffed animal? Did you play with certain animal toys? Have you been bitten by an animal? Are you allergic to cats or bee stings? Can you recall a specific incidence from childhood where an animal played a significant role? Was there a movie or fairy tale with a certain animal that influenced you as a child?

When we fear an animal, it is usually in our life to teach us valuable lessons. For example, spiders can be a writing totem. If you fear them, you may need to write a book, or it may be therapeutic to keep a journal to process your feelings. Possibly you are an avid reader or will learn much through the written word. Maybe you will seek a profession that uses words to teach others. When we use the gifts of the animal, the fear may lessen or dissolve. The totem that is feared can completely transform an area of our life.

It is possible to love an animal that is a birth totem and to have a fearful encounter. Perhaps wolf is a birth totem, and as an adolescent you were bitten by a dog. The bite can serve to get your attention. Fear-inducing situations also act as a kind of test. It is a type of initiation and a call to realize the powerful energy of the animal.

Other totem animals will show up in our life to work with us during a specific time period. Some may work with us for a relationship or a project. Animals may come to bring specific messages or guidance. They can show up and help us with difficult passages in our lives. Loved ones who have passed into the spirit realm may temporarily take the form of an animal. Once an animal comes to us and is recognized, an animal as totem may stay with us forever. Others come temporarily to teach a lesson, provide guidance, or give a message.

How do we know if the house wren singing at our kitchen window is bringing us a message? And how do we interpret the meanings of their appearance or understand the message?

Animals that are totems or that bring messages will always catch your attention. They may be in an unusual place. They may do something that makes you pause and take notice. They may literally put themselves in front of you or come into your house. They may get your attention by being a nuisance or making noise.

The willingness to communicate with nature and the animal world is the first step to understanding messages and guidance. When we invite animal connection and communication, it opens the door to their world, and our intuition and knowing will sharpen. Nature's language is one of symbolism, and often it is a matter of making symbolic connections.

To help interpret the meanings of messages, ask yourself a series of questions:

- What type of animal has come to you?
- What are the patterns of its behavior in nature?
- What is it doing that caught your attention?
- How does the animal symbolically relate to what is currently going on in your life?
- What is the animal's strength or weakness and how does it apply to you?
- How did this encounter initially make you feel?

As we begin to have encounters and allow our instincts to develop naturally, it will get easier to know what messages or guidance we are receiving. It is a process that requires love, trust, and patience. But nature is generous and will reward you greatly.

It is extremely important to acknowledge animal totems with gratitude and appreciation. Thanking animals that come to us will bring more encounters. There are numerous ways to acknowledge totems and express gratitude. Sincerely saying the words "thank you" sends the frequency of gratitude out into nature. We can acknowledge totems by displaying images of them in our homes or gardens. We can make monetary donations to animal organizations. We can volunteer our time at animal shelters or sanctuaries. We can maintain a backyard bird feeder, have a garden, or plant flowers and trees that support wildlife. Find creative ways to respect, appreciate, and coexist with the natural world, and you will be gifted a hundredfold in return.

A TRUE STORY

The hawk has been a totem of mine for a very long time. Hawk protects me, guides me, and gives me messages. My father often comes to me in the form of hawk.

Shortly after my father passed away, he appeared to me in a dream. In the dream, he led me by the hand and took me outside to the stone steps in our back yard. He said that he loved me and told me to take care of my mother. He told me to go there, to those steps in the yard, and that he would be there. And then, before my eyes, he faded away. In the dream, I began to cry, and my crying woke me.

Awake, I scrambled from my bed and ran out the back door to the stone steps. I stood there, fresh from the dream, with intense longing in my heart, and called for him. A shadow crossed over me, and when I looked up, a huge hawk was circling above my head. He was flying low and I saw as he bent his head and looked down at me. He swooped down lower and flew toward me as I reached up for him. I knew this was my father.

From that day on, hawk became an important totem and has been there for me throughout my life. He has come to me in times of joy and life-changing events. He was there for the birth of my children and has continued to watch over them. He has come in times of crisis and need. Hawk comes when I think of my father, and when I call to him for guidance or protection.

Decades later, when my mother was dying, hawk was there. She was in the hospital for five days. Every morning, I took the same route in to the hospital. And every morning, as if he was waiting for me, I saw a huge red-tailed hawk. He sat on a telephone pole that was close to a red light, and as I slowed my car, he would bend his head to me. On day four, sitting on the very next pole, was one crow. The hawk bent his head to me, but the crow looked away, off into the distance. On that day, my mother took a turn for the worse. On the fifth morning, the hawk wasn't there, and she died that day. I knew then that my father had been waiting for her.

After I wrote those last lines, I sat for a long while remembering. Then I wondered, How do I finish this story? Do I just leave it there? What else is there to say?

And then I asked myself a serious question: "Do I even want to tell this story?" My attention was drawn immediately to a pair of framed, black-and-white photographs I keep above my desk. One is of my grandmother (my father's mother) standing by an old vehicle, her pet crow perched on the car's roof. Next to that, my father as a young man, before the war. He is kneeling beside his dog, one hand on the beagle's head, the other hand gently on the dog's chest. The love between them is apparent. Yes, these photographs seemed to be saying. Yes, go ahead and tell it.

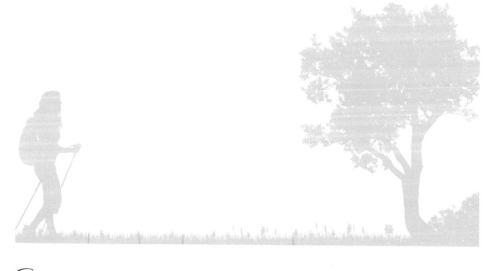

~ AFTERWORD ~

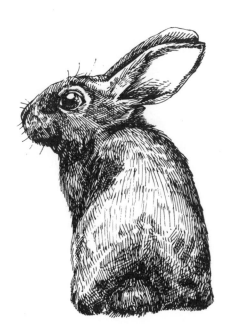

The woman who follows the crowd will usually go no further than the crowd.
The woman who walks alone is likely to find herself
in places no one has ever been before.
—Albert Einstein

About a year into the writing of my *Soul Stepping* book, my daughter, Rosie, sent me a gift. It was a little book titled *How to Walk* by Thich Nhat Hanh. Before the title page, she wrote, "For inspiration! On this project and the next ..." Such an optimist.

Throughout history, there have been a great many sages who have walked for inspiration. Many have walked to connect with nature, God, and themselves. For instance, Henry David Thoreau and John Muir wrote extensively about walking, almost as if walking was their religion or a necessary lifeline to their sanity.

And there *is* a spiritual greatness that can be harnessed through walking. On a practical level, walking is the best method I know to quickly and effectively shift negative energy or rid yourself of unwanted negative emotions. But walking can give you so much more.

This book should help you find what you need, when you need it. It is my hope that by soul stepping, you will open or deepen your connection to nature, your spirit, and your source. My wish for you is that you will begin to cultivate a trust for yourself and your own inner soul wisdom. It is my dream that every single one of us will step on Mother Earth with reverence and love.

For your own inspiration, I leave you with the first words in the little book my daughter gave to me. In his book *How to Walk*, Thich Nhat Hanh begins by writing "The first thing to do is to lift your foot" (Nhat Hahn 2015).

~ACKNOWLEDGMENTS~

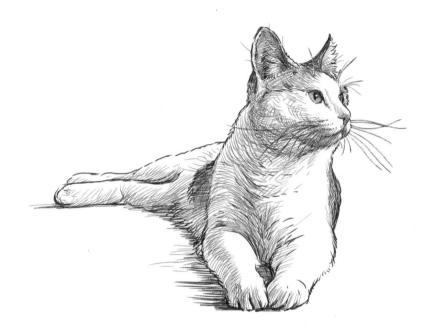

First we crawl. Then we walk.

There are no adequate words to express my deep and endless gratitude to my daughter, Rosie. I have a personal policy that no major writing project of mine goes out into the world until she reads it first. She was my cheerleader from beginning to end. I sent her pages and chapters, and as always, her real gift to me is her honesty. She is brilliant, a professor no less. And, although it is not her profession, she beautifully performed the role of a firm and critical first editor. Thank you, Rosie.

Great gratitude to my editor, Dinah Roseberry, for her original interest in this book. She answered all my questions with speed, humor, and skill. She had answers before I could even form my questions. I am especially grateful for her keen ability to tamp down anxiety and replace it with a feeling of ease. And she made me laugh. It was Dinah's contagious spirit of fearlessness that truly walked this project to the end. Thank you, Dinah.

~BIBLIOGRAPHY~

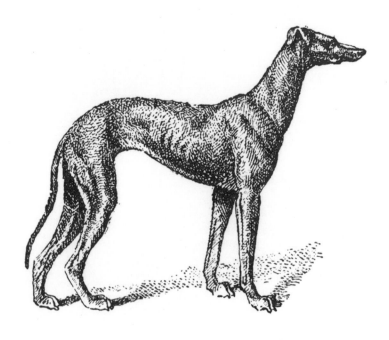

Eden, Donna, with David Feinstein. *Energy Medicine: Balancing Your Body's Energy for Optimal Health, Joy, and Vitality.* New York: Jeremy P. Tarcher / Penguin Group, 2008.

Freke, Timothy. *Rumi Wisdom: Daily Teachings from the Great Sufi Master.* New York: Sterling, 2000.

Hicks, Ester, and Jerry Hicks. *Ask and It Is Given: Learning to Manifest Your Desires.* Carlsbad, CA: Hay House, 2004.

Lamott, Anne. *Traveling Mercies: Some Thoughts on Faith.* New York: Anchor Books, 1999.

Nhat Hanh, Thich. *How to Walk.* Berkeley, CA: Parallax, 2015.

Ober, Clinton, Stephen T. Sinatra, and Martin Zucker. *Earthing: The Most Important Health Discovery Ever!* Laguna Beach, CA: Basic Health Publications, 2004.

Vitale, Joe, and Ihaleakala Hew Len. *Zero Limits: The Secret Hawaiian System for Wealth, Health, Peace, and More.* Hoboken, NJ: John Wiley & Sons, 2007.

SUGGESTED READING LIST

Andrews, Ted. *Animal Speak: The Spiritual & Magical Powers of Creatures Great & Small*. St. Paul, MN: Llewellyn, 1994. (Any book by Ted Andrews. Always.)

Eden, Donna, with Dondi Dahlin. *The Little Book of Energy Medicine: The Essential Guide to Balancing Your Body's Energies*. New York: Penguin Group, 2012. (Any book by Donna Eden.)

Emoto, Masaru. *The Hidden Messages of Water*. Translated by David A. Thayne. Hillsboro, OR: Beyond Words, 2004.

Hay, Louise L., *You Can Heal Your Life*. Carlsbad, CA: Hay House, 1999. (Any book by Louise Hay.)

Hicks, Ester, and Jerry Hicks. *The Law of Attraction: The Basics of the Teachings of Abraham*. Carlsbad, CA: Hay House, 2006. (Any book by Ester and Jerry Hicks.)

Kabat-Zinn, Jon. *Wherever You Go, There You Are: Mindfulness Meditation in Everyday Life*. New York: Hyperion, 1994.

Reilly, Harrold J., and Ruth Hagy Brod. *The Edgar Cayce Handbook for Health through Drugless Therapy*. New York: A.R.E. Press, 1975.

Shinn, Florence Scovel. *The Writings of Florence Scovel Shinn*. Camarillo, CA: DeVorss, 1996.

Stearn, Jess. *Edgar Cayce: The Sleeping Prophet*. New York: Bantam Books, 1967.

Stearn, Jess. *Yoga, Youth, and Reincarnation: A Modern Step-by-Step Approach to the Ancient Art of Yoga*. New York: Bantam Books, 1968.

Turner, Gladys Davis, and Mae Gimbert St. Clair. *Individual Reference File of Extracts from the Edgar Cayce Readings*. Virginia Beach, VA: Edgar Cayce Foundation, 1976.

~ INDEX ~

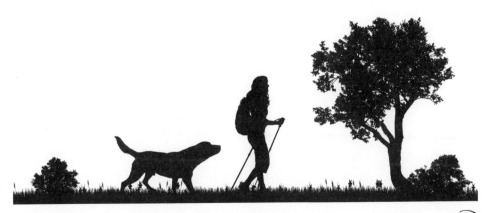

~ ABOUT THE AUTHOR ~

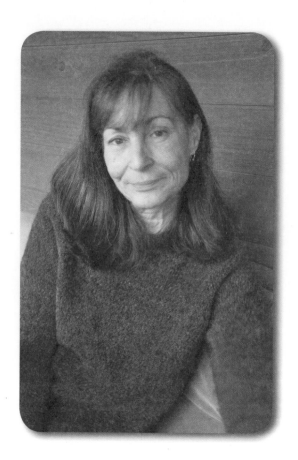

Ann Trump is an author, artist, and diviner, as well as a Feng Shui practitioner, and is trained as a massage therapist in the Edgar Cayce / Dr. Harrold J. Reilly method. She is skilled in diverse areas of divination, including Tarot and casting stones. An expert in nature signs, she is also a gifted animal interpreter. Ann is cocreator, illustrator, and coauthor of *The Saint Deck* and *The Saint Deck Book*. She lives in rural Pennsylvania.